Younger Next Decade

After Fifty, the Transitional Decade,

and What You Need to Know

Younger Next Decade

After Fifty, the Transitional Decade,

and What You Need to Know

by Barbara Ebel, M.D.

ISBN: 978-0-9829351-5-6

For all of us over fifty.

May the rest of our journey be trouble free.

We realize now what older generations

knew before us: we are simply young

people born earlier.

Chapter 1
Introduction

Every book begins with page one. You and I are going to start fresh, especially if you just had your fiftieth birthday or if that *big one* is looming just ahead. Please consider that your fiftieth birthday is a mile marker in your life and that the next ten years - what we'll call your transitional decade - will fundamentally set the stage for how you decide to live the rest of your life.

Also, introductions are in order. Instead of you getting to the end of this book and reading "about the author," I'm giving you a short scoop from the get-go. First, I'm an author and have multiple published works, including multiple genres. But here's the thing - not only am I a physician - but I try whole-heartedly every day to practice what I preach by incorporating what I'm about to tell you into my lifestyle. I, too, am only human, and you can strive to be perfect, but don't come down on yourself too hard if you can't live up to ideal lifestyle standards all of the time. What I'm going to do here is to give you some insight into the why and how of living smarter after fifty. After all, we are simply young people born earlier.

Second, since conciseness is a big thing with me, I am going to try my best to deliver advice as succinctly as possible. Since we're multitasking and leading busy lives, time is a precious commodity. Heck, actually, we need to talk about that later. My goal is also to make this a *fun* read. It's a turn-off to be preached to. I want to supplement what your family doctor may or may not tell you and I want to add to all the other information you read, believe, don't believe, fail to follow, or are as stubborn as a mule to incorporate into your life. I hope to give you some brand new ideas. We're going to make this enjoyable, we're going to do it together, and I'm going to deliver some fresh approaches.

Third, if you're clicking page turns on an eBook reader you may not see this; if you have a paperback, then you may have noticed it already. There will be more than one chapter titled *Spirit.* No. It has nothing to do with spirituality or religion, although perhaps you could argue that underneath my philosophy, spiritualism has to do with its foundation. Whether you are religious or not, I will lay the cards on the table and tell you I have no right or background to give you a spiel with religious overtones. My *Spirit* chapters have to do with a feeling and a love for being alive.

If you've hit that milestone birthday and are becoming increasingly unhappy when you look in the mirror, here's a fact that the infomercials and the big cosmetic companies won't be too pleased about. Those crow's feet popping out around your eyes, and those baby vertical lines sprouting from your upper lip, and those puffy lower lids aren't erased by the contents in a bottle.

However, there are good products out there that help subdue those budding features but don't deplete your bank account for them. You can find appropriately priced products which have the latest dermatological ingredients for revitalizing and moisturizing your skin, including scrubs and exfoliants. I went on a medical mission several years ago to Mexico and, lo and behold, was I surprised to find Retin-A tubes of varying concentrations - non-prescription and dirt cheap - on drug store shelves. Many of you know that Retin-A is the ingredient of some high-end commercial products advertised to slow skin aging. I bought a bag of tubes and I'm still occasionally smearing a light film on at bedtime.

So, yes, there are some products that help your skin look refreshed, but as we all know, or should know, the Hollywood women who "look so good," and "haven't aged at all," probably have a preferred plastic surgeon for facelifts, forehead lifts,

blepharoplasties, cheek implants, rhinoplasties, a tuck here or a tuck there, and a large chest double curvature. Even easier than those, are all the injectable prescription botulinum toxin products such as Botox, Dysport, and Javederm. Injections with these products can help camouflage facial wrinkles and are becoming as routine for some people as a once or twice a year formal dental exam; not to mention teeth whitening.

Do you remember American history which incorporated beliefs from our founding fathers? The generation reading this was taught straight factual American history as a subject way back then, just like they were taught cursive, a soon-to-be archaic means to communicate, because it seems to be on its way out. All you'll have to do in the future is type. (I hope younger people practice a signature however; they may need it in the transitional decade to sign a credit card slip for anti-aging cream).

I digress. Here's my history. Juan Ponce de León y Figueroa was the Spanish explorer who led the first European expedition to the state of Florida, which he named. He was looking for the Fountain of Youth. Well, he didn't find it. Today, there are more older people in Florida than ever, and they look pretty weathered to me. I've done the living in Florida thing, too, so I'm not picking on them. It's just that I'll have something to say about the sun. But right now I do have something more to say about the Fountain of Youth.

Here's the thing. Or here's my bright idea founded on sound principle. And I am a firm believer in new ideas, which usually take some time to accept. As a matter of fact, one of my favorite Albert Einstein quotes is *"If at first the idea is not absurd, then there is not hope for it."* The Fountain of Youth is not to be found in a jar or in a sink hole. It's going to be found in the laboratory.

Chapter 2
Spirit

Since this is so important, *spirit* is next. But first, I don't want to leave you wondering about the tantalizing ending to the previous chapter. I'm trying to make it exciting for those addicted thriller/suspense/mass-marketed paperback readers. Yes, I'm talking about you *guys*.

For those of us in the transitional decade, we have seen technological change at the speed of light. Even more so, think of the change a forty-year-old has seen. The high tech world has sped up even faster during their lifetime than ours because our earlier years were more laid back and life moved at a slower pace.

If you think back to the historic day in December 1980 when John Lennon was assassinated outside his New York apartment, there was no live television coverage with a hovering helicopter at the police scene, we didn't receive an instantaneous text message from a friend or a news source, and word of mouth didn't spread like wildfire from cell phones stuck to our ears. In the U.S., the announcement came from Howard Cosell, after the shooting was ABC's judgment call to break the news during a New England Patriots and Miami Dolphins football game. Announcer Cosell finally told us of the "unspeakable tragedy" that Lennon had been shot twice and had died en-route to Roosevelt Hospital. Jump ahead to today and we are bombarded with news from multiple sources as it's happening.

So what is the point? Molecular biologists, scientific institutions, and gene researchers continue to unravel our understanding of chromosomes down to the very ends of our double-stranded DNA. Think of boat ropes which are perfectly cut and intact at their ends. Over time, the end starts to fray and come apart which is also occurring at the tail ends of your chromosomes. These end points are called telomeres. Although the telomeres try to prevent the rest of the chromosomes from getting shorter, they can lose a bit themselves with cell division and stress. Importantly for this discussion, telomeres play a part in aging. Except for sperm and egg cells, cells die when the telomeres become excessively short, and herein lies the link with the aging process. Telomeres that have aged and are shortening too much correlate with the changes we see with aging.

Aging cells are associated with shorter telomeres but there is a more abundant enzyme called telomerase in egg and sperm cells which actually help add length to telomeres, which in turn adds longer life to a cell. Now, at the basis of brilliant discoveries and ideas there is simplicity. The Fountain of Youth may lie in manipulating the ends of telomeres to keep them from fraying. Perhaps that can be done with the knowledge we have regarding telomerase or something like chromosomal super glue which adheres only to the telomeres' specific nucleic acid bases. But don't take it from me; it's the dedicated researchers who spend their lives piecing together their analysis for our benefit.

We are living in a world driven by technological advancement that was unthinkable early on in our lifetime. Gene and genomics research is the next big thing. Preventing the aging process is fraught with wonderful and horrific possibilities, but probably what's going to happen is something in between. Maybe in the next century, I would not be writing a book called *Younger Next Decade; After Fifty,* but writing a book called *Younger Next Decade; After One Hundred!*

It's okay to be optimistic about methods available today to help you look younger, but those are band-aids compared to what's looming ahead.

Now that we've put our cold creams, chemical peels, and retin-A aside for the moment, let's talk about something much more fundamental. Let's get to the root of existence. It was my husband who came up with the word *spirit*. The word surfaced not while I was discussing this book; he used it to describe one of our dogs.

I might as well tell you right now that I plan on talking about dogs later. They are so important that I actually devote half of a medical lecture I present to residents on dogs. But I digress again. My husband and I have dogs, one of which is a Chesapeake Bay retriever named Chester. He's a therapy dog, the star of a children's book series, and my children say he's so smart, "it's scary." A few days ago, we started out the day like usual. We got ready to walk and Chester sprinted around the house with a couch pillow that has become his. He politely ran up and down the hallway and whenever he stopped and waited, he placed the pillow between his paws and sank his muzzle perfectly on top of it. It's always obvious he thinks better than to rest his canine head on the wooden floor.

These kind of antics progressed. We left the house with all the dogs and walked the empty country roads with woods flanking us on both sides. Chester, who is unleashed, sprinted a short distance into the woods to do his business. On his emergence, he grabbed a stick and rushed over to present it to us. He dropped it at our feet and then coaxed me to dig a carrot out of my pocket for him, but then darted off again to taunt a deer who watched us with curiosity. If the weather is cool, then Chester's motions are exaggerated, and his energy seems to pop from a bottle. This particular day I watched with my usual fondness but blabbered my appreciation of him to my husband. "He's so happy - his tail never stops – he still has the exact enthusiasm he had his first year - he still plays like a puppy."

I went on with my descriptions about Chester and then added. "You know, he's seven and a half, and with big dogs, the equivalent of one dog year is similar to seven human years and more. Actually, he's coming up to about my age. Fifty-eight. And look at him."

My husband mulled this over and said. "He's got *spirit.*" Yes, that's how this smart dog is living his whole life – with *spirit.*

The perfect word. My husband hit the head of the nail. If we humans carry a vitality and an enthusiasm for life, and an understanding of this gift called life, and if we experience our existence as much as possible with a positive outlook and joy; well, I think that's called *spirit.*

Have you ever noticed the difference between someone's attitude who's living life to the fullest versus someone who is just going through the everyday motions? I noticed it with my own mother. As she grew older, she became more socially active and independent. Into her seventies and eighties she looked more gorgeous than ever. She actually looked older in her fifties. Her spirit had developed and everyone around her saw and felt it.

Now, just another word. You may be saying. "Sure, that's easy in principle, but you can't have spirit when you have a half-dozen big problems on your plate." You are partially correct about that. But take it from someone who's been told "you've been through hell and back." Life does have its ups-and-downs. Do everything you can to weather those times - purposeful distractions got me through - and remember that inside you is a fundamental spirit that no one can take away that you must take every opportunity to flourish. Water yourself like a rose, from *inside.*

Chapter 3
Smoking

You smokers out there are probably tired of the non-smokers picking on you. Smoke-free workplaces, restaurants, and public places are clamping down on what you believe is your right to smoke.

Let's put that issue aside because we're not here to debate personal rights. Think of this book as a mantra to self improvement in this critical transitional decade where our bodies are trying to catapult us into changes which will put us closer to death. You see, our bodies do that anyway, but by the way we live in modern society, we are hastening that process by inflicting unnecessary ills on our organ systems.

Why do I call it the transitional decade? Our body's peak performance declines in our thirties. We hear it all the time. The stellar athletes we know about, whether football players, famous pro-golfers or Olympic medalists, "retire" in their thirties. We saw their awe-inspiring performances; but then, no matter how much they train, they can't repeat those gold medal times or bodily maneuvers again. Every now and then, there's an exception, but Rocky's fourth sequel just isn't the same as when he jabbed and punched into thin air while running up the steps to the Philadelphia Museum of Art. We just can't will our bodies to perform as they did when we were eighteen or twenty five.

Here's super good news and you'll hear it again: Normal aging is not so much to blame for the functional losses between our peak thirties, later adult forties, and our senior sixties. What makes the biggest difference to our health and decline are *disorders*. And many disorders beckon us because of our lifestyle!

So, first I'm going to talk about your pulmonary system or lungs, and along with that, tobacco use. You can't escape it because I am a physician. Also, just because you can't see something, doesn't mean it doesn't exist. Or, as they say, if a tree falls in a forest, did it make noise even though you weren't there? Smoker's lungs look like a blackened air filter you would pull out from under your car hood. Just because you can't see inside your chest, that doesn't mean you should pretend that your lungs haven't been damaged.

Cilia sweep mucus and unnatural substances from your respiratory passages. They are tiny and hair-like, but cigarette smoke impairs their function. For Pete's sake, clean up the air pockets and breathing channels, please, by not smoking.

Here are the normal physiologic pulmonary changes we undergo as we age. Our lungs lose elasticity or compliance. There is less flexibility when the lungs fill with air and return to their original size or shape. There is less vital capacity and an increased residual volume. After your thirty- year-old lung took a breath, it would deflate and empty out like a balloon. Now your lungs deflate but do not remove all the air – there's a volume of air that just sits there because they have become less elastic. That volume now goes unused for the proper exchange of air – or oxygen.

We could go on about that, but the point is for you to have more of an understanding of why, as we age, we become increasingly short of breath when exercising, especially after periods without regular activity. Also, as we age, we stand a greater morbidity risk if we come down with pneumonia or a pulmonary disorder. So let's not give outside forces or more ammunition to Mother Nature to age us sooner than she should.

In the past, I have had patients tell me, "A doctor told me once I have COPD," and when I inquired further, they confessed they don't know what that is. Sometimes they recall an initial discussion about it in their doctor's office, but the brief insight into the problem didn't stick. They ended up with a diagnosis and go without follow-up visits, they move, change doctors, and fail to ever understand or get a grip about their disease.

COPD stands for chronic obstructive pulmonary disease. It means your lungs are abnormal, and they are abnormal in this case because of their normal response to a nasty toxin which is cigarette smoke. So, I'm telling you that cigarette smoking is the primary risk factor for COPD, and COPD is a progressive disease which makes you symptom-laden and old before your time.

Many of you have heard of bronchitis (chronic obstructive bronchitis) and emphysema. Each one is a variant of COPD and smokers usually have features of both.

You can officially be diagnosed with the obstructive bronchitis variant if your cough is productive for a minimum of three months in two years. The "obstructive" part means, like a clogged pipe, airflow is hindered. You can probably identify the heavy smoker sitting next to you at church or at a meeting. They seem to be always clearing the mucous which is irritating their breathing passages.

With emphysema, there is actually destruction of lung tissue. It's like finding holes in a car's air filter. Parts of lung tissue can collapse, and other areas can hyperinflate – the lung tissue just doesn't know what to do with itself with all that steamy smoke blowing around in there.

There are other causes of COPD. But the biggest risk factor is cigarette smoking which causes your lung tissue to mount an inflammatory response, and then it's all downhill. If you are in your forties and fifties, you are a smoker, and you quite often have a productive cough, you're on your way.

Are you getting more short of breath? That's called dyspnea. You can show how smart you are by knowing that word, which can help camouflage the fact that you're not being too bright by smoking! Yes, I'm being hard on you, but you say it's only a book.

Please consider this a sincere attempt to help you live longer. Do yourself a favor by quitting the habit right now.

Here are just a few more things to help you with your decision. And it is a decision. If you continue to smoke, by your late fifties the pulmonary infection you get will be a lot worse. Your chances of getting other associated disorders and cancer are greater. You have a much greater risk of heart and pulmonary problems going hand in hand, and as your lungs worsen, your body will be getting less and less oxygen. You've seen skinny elderly men and women with oxygen tubing dangling from their nostrils, sitting in wheelchairs. Oh yes, the muscle wasting comes with the territory, too. Do you want to increase your chances of ending up like that?

I wouldn't be telling you this if there wasn't hope for you to stop smoking. If you quit, the progression of any lung disease will slow. It may not stop all together, but imagine how bad it would be if you continue. My mother smoked almost a pack a day until her fifties. Over time she tapered down to a cigarette or two a day, and then finally quit by sixty. She lived to 85 and died of non-pulmonary problems.

Quitting smoking is no easy chore. You may have tried but gave in to the addiction again. You have to work on your mind, and until you can convince yourself you are going to do it, it's practically impossible. That's why behavior modification is so important. Get help from a therapist or a smoker's group.

Also, your family practitioner or internal medicine practitioner can play a role. Ask about weaning off smoking by using nicotine replacement methods. Have you heard of electronic or e-cigarettes? They are meant to help you simulate the act of smoking and will produce an inhaled mist. There are also good prescription medications that your doctor can prescribe.

Here's my solution. Don't reject this idea until you've given it some hard thought. And, consider again my most loved quote by Albert Einstein: "*If at first the idea is not absurd, then there is not hope for it."* Use a little psychology on your mind. Instead of, "I have to quit. I can't smoke," make the following an absolute rule not to be broken under any circumstance:

"I cannot raise a cigarette to my lips."

You can do it. I know you can.

Chapter 4
Diet and Weight

I can't (and I won't) discuss these two topics separately. They go together like cheeseburgers and French fries.

Yes, that's funny, but not as funny as when you start replacing your clothes because they're too tight, or you look in a full length mirror and feel uncomfortable at what you see. You tell yourself you'll start cutting back calories, but the next day you have a decent size lunch and later, you're invited to a friend's for dinner where you chow down with everyone else, and then come home to carrot cake sitting on the counter. You feel deprived because you never had an adequate dessert all day, so you plunge into that as well. The next day, you look in the mirror and say to yourself you'll have to start cutting back. However, you make chocolate chip cookies because your daughter is coming to visit over the weekend. You must sample them while they're still warm, and they are gone in two days - well before she pulls into the driveway.

Does that sound like you? If not, then perhaps it wasn't the carrot cake you longed for, but a big tray of peach cobbler with ice cream or a family-size bag of sea-salted potato chips.

That's why you can't separate one from the other. Inappropriate eating habits lead to weight gain... and bad eating habits and weight gain during your transitional decade are going to lead to the *disorders* which make you older than your time. Disorders like adult onset diabetes or hypertension or cardiovascular disease.

We are all aware of the weight problem in the United States. If you get a newspaper or receive online newslinks then you read the statistics often enough, and I won't bore you with those staggering obesity statistics. You even know that this obesity has filtered down to our children. It had to sooner or later, because a family's eating habits involve the entire household. Don't you often see a large mother, large father and a chubby child walking down the supermarket aisle together? On the other hand, you see trim parents along a hiking trail with their lean children, and you can bet the parents pay attention to the food they all eat.

To drive my point home, how about watching a three set DVD documentary which is enjoyable, enlightening, and has spectacular footage? In and of itself, it's a well-deserved addition to anyone's DVD library. It is the BBC's *The Human Planet*. They spent years filming this in the most remote and rarely, or never filmed parts of the earth, and it highlights man's daily life in natural environments. (Although, to our partial dislike, they have a section called *"Cities."*).

The Human Planet's three discs include episodes on *Oceans, Deserts, Arctic, Jungles, Mountains, Grasslands, Rivers,* and *Cities.* The human beings in the far reaching parts of the globe which exist in these filmed geographic locations didn't know it, but they all have something in common. No one is overweight. Most of the storyline centers around where and how they attain their next meals. Whether it was the father and son training and bringing their hawks out to hunt a small grassland mammal for their dinner; or a bare-footed father dangerously scaling to a jungle treetop to scoop out a honeycomb despite the bees' aggressive stings; or the unarmed African men who courageously walk right into a lion pack feasting on their kill to take the grizzled meat themselves - these are amazing insights into human beings eating to live and not living to eat.

What was most disturbing were the activities of a group of children. Still hungry after their family's provisions, their *play* was also their own hunt as they scooped sticks into holes and took risks grabbing tarantulas. This pulls at your heartstrings to watch them forage for something so dangerous in order to have a snack. They built their own fire and roasted them like we would roast marshmallows and stick s'mores in our mouths. However, as far as their spirit, they seemed as happy, or more, as an American kid eating Twinkies and playing Nintendo.

Obviously, this is not the way we would like to see any child obtain their next bite to eat. Yet many of us have gone to the other extreme. We don't do anything for our meal except purchase it and shove it down our throats.

If you really want to drive home this psychological message on what we've become and how we can alter it, then watch one of the above DVD's and then walk through your grocery store. Mostly what you see and grab are boxes of every size and shape, and bottles of every size and shape. Processed, boxed, canned, and bagged food are everywhere. So are put-together frozen "dinners," and other frozen ready-made poultry, pizzas, waffles and egg biscuits. How much trouble is it anyway to boil a three-minute fresh egg, or open a healthy container of yogurt, or cut up some lettuce, tomatoes, onions, and avocado and make a smart salad?

So what is it with us? Have we gotten so fat that's it's too much trouble to open the refrigerator to pull out ingredients, scramble some eggs, peel an orange, and slide bread in the toaster? Instead, we have to open a waffle box, put it in the microwave, and saturate that thawed cardboard-tasting breakfast with butter?

If you're starting to feel uncomfortable, that's good. Please don't get annoyed at the messenger, however. I'd like you to start changing how you see things so you alter your behavior and stick with the changes.

Now wait, you say. You are around fifty years old and working forty hours a week, running a neighborhood committee, running back and forth to see the college kids or having them home every few weekends, and many nights you want to sit down to watch the newest DVD release. Where's the time to cook? It is so much easier to pop that fast food in the car on the way home or throw that frozen dinner in the microwave.

First, a healthy meal doesn't have to consume your time. It probably won't take any longer than diverting to the drive-through window and then waiting in line. Think about throwing some ingredients into a crock pot in the morning; it will be ready when you get home. I even throw old fashioned five-minute oatmeal in a crock pot in the morning for one hour, freeing me up to do other things.

Second, even if you don't like to cook, there are plenty of ways to get around that. Always have yogurt and fruit around. Mix them together. How about regular vanilla yogurt? I mention vanilla yogurt because supermarket yogurt is now also getting trashed with artificial sweeteners and candy cups on top with chocolate chips. Buy salads (yes, get bagged if you're that busy), canned tuna fish, and even canned chicken. Have you ever tried mixing low fat mayonnaise with honey, celery, cranberries, pecans and yellow raisins with canned chicken? However, if you have more time, buy a roasted chicken and skin and shred that instead. You must get my drift by now. Stock up on some appropriate cookbooks for easy but healthy preparations. There are dozens out there.

Quit making excuses for eating too much and the wrong things.

Now that I've pointed some things out so you're not shocked at my guidelines for this chapter, here you go:

Diet and Weight Guidelines:

Don't eat anything passed through a window!

Don't eat anything that wasn't available 100 years ago!

———

If you are committed to change and stay on track for the transitional decade and beyond, then the first guideline "Don't eat anything passed through a window," is easier than "Don't eat anything that wasn't available 100 years ago." Still, I'm putting them out there. You wanted some good sound advice, didn't you? You know your body's metabolism isn't going to handle the same calories it did before, right? In the transitional decade, men should decrease their caloric intake by approximately 33% of what it was when they were eighteen years old if all other things are equal; for women, it's about 25%.

We could label the above as rules instead of guidelines, but there would be exceptions to the rules. One-hundred-years ago people commonly used lard, which is pig's fat. They used it as a cooking shortening and spread it like butter. Certainly common sense is needed for both guidelines; they should serve you well in most instances.

Maybe you have previously stayed at a normal, steady weight - but that won't happen anymore in the transitional decade if you start slipping into the bad habits of most Americans. There are more than twice the number of us in the transitional decade who are obese than when we were twenty.

Obesity is a less rigid term for excess body fat, so if you want to get down to brass tacks, look up your BMI. That means Body Mass Index and it's calculated by dividing your weight by height along with other numbers. It's the real index of your body size because it does consider weight plus height. Just Google BMI and you'll find BMI quick calculators where you can plug in your numbers. Make sure you use a site with a BMI graph where you can see where you really stand. Your BMI will fit into one of the following areas of the graph: underweight, normal range, overweight, and obese. Consider your BMI and graph finding your absolute scale. It won't lie to you or allow you to make excuses about your weight because you're so tall.

We'll talk about exercise later, because I want to separate it and give it its own spotlight. For right now, linking diet and weight together, or *overweight* together, helps me stress one more thing.

You can exercise all you want, but the primary key to weight loss and maintenance is your daily calorie count. If you keep lumping butter on that bread instead of one pat of butter or low fat butter, it's going to show up on your thighs, your flabby arms, or your beer belly.

There are plenty of diets available just like there are decent quick and easy, healthy cookbook recipes. You see or read the following all the time, but here it is again. Like purchasing a book, sometimes you have to see it up to ten times before you buy the idea or buy the product.

Make sure you include a variety of foods every day from the major food groups. Ones that you like. Are there vegetables and fruit, lean protein and whole grains, and low fat dairy products in your grocery cart? Get some tasty nuts and seeds. Sometimes you don't have the time to cut up a cauliflower or sometimes the vegetables you like aren't seasonal. Bagged frozen vegetables are an easy and healthy way to get your vegetable vitamins. That's what microwaves are for besides warming coffee, especially because now you're going to decrease the frequency of zapping greasy popcorn in there. Here's where I really promote frozen broccoli. Broccoli is on every wholesome food list and there's no excuse to not stock up your freezer with this healthy, inexpensive, and noteworthy green vegetable.

A special word about carbohydrates. Most of us love them. Besides the vegetables, make sure whole wheat or whole grains are included in your bread, cereal, oatmeal, pasta and wild or brown rice.

Now, taper the amount you eat because even if it's healthy food, any excess in is going to turn to yellow fat globules underneath your skin. It's not a pretty sight in the OR when a surgeon has to get into the abdominal cavity or leg of someone obese.

Just think how much less food you'd consume in a month if you controlled every portion you eat. Another trick is to eat more small meals a day to prevent too much hunger from setting in. But limiting your calories to less than 1200 a day isn't going to last, although for a few initial days it can be the jump start to a real weight loss commitment. Check with an M.D. or a nutritionist if you're unsure about launching into a diet. If you have a significant medical history, also see your doctor so your diet plan can be supervised or you can receive further advice.

Now here's something most people don't know about regarding weight. We don't usually know the deep information of other people's professions or trades – things that they spend years learning or then practicing. For instance, I wouldn't have a clue how to clear a mine shaft, or bait a running swordfish line in the Atlantic, or know the complexities of just one person's job at NASA. So here's the scoop: I am an anesthesiologist. If you need an elective surgery, or worse yet, an emergency surgery and you are morbidly obese or overweight with a preponderance of pounds around your chest, neck and lower face, you could give your anesthesiologist a severe panic attack.

I exaggerate the panic attack because a well-trained anesthesiologist should remain calm - but he or she is going to sweat bullets and perhaps use every airway trick in his or her armament to try and secure your airway. In essence, you are at a much greater risk with your airway protection if your normal human being anatomy has expanded like a frog's vocal sac. Do you know that for a significant surgery, an anesthesiologist must place a breathing tube down your throat, and the ease of doing so depends on multiple factors? It's too complicated to go through. Suffice to say it takes years to master difficult airways, but it doesn't mean all airway problems can be solved. Securing your airway means you're able to breathe and that, in translation, means your life. Please don't be more of a medical emergency because of your size than the surgical procedure you've shown up for!

As I've mentioned, by not watching your weight and diet, you may gain a disorder which will cause your cells to age a lot quicker. I won't talk about disorders for the time being. We'll tackle them together later in the book.

Let's get back to something so much more uplifting – spirit.

I've only said the guidelines twice, so don't forget, and please think seriously about using them:

Don't eat anything passed through a window.

Don't eat anything that wasn't available 100 years ago.

Chapter 5
Spirit

Since Chapter 2, have you been kindling your *spirit*? Unless you have already found your inner sanctum, we have work to do.

During the transitional decade some of you may be retiring. It doesn't have to happen in your sixties if you've planned for it early instead. Perhaps you are semi-retired or not working. Easing into retirement is the best of all worlds; it helps you collect ideas about hobbies and activities you are going to pursue and begin dabbling in them. But before you go ahead with a bigger list of things to do, even though pleasurable, let's focus on relaxation. Mental relaxation. Then, we're going to talk about mental productivity. I think both of these things are fundamental to your spirit.

I once had a few sessions with a counselor when stress was so overwhelming that I felt like I was carrying around the load from a heavy cement truck. Most mental health workers - psychiatrists, psychologists, and therapists - take a "you talk, I listen" approach. This man knew he couldn't do anything for me in the normal sense because unless my problem went away, he couldn't pull me from my hole. Now, if you know many physician personalities at all, you know they fill the Type A personality box quite nicely. So as he veered off to teach me relaxation techniques, the skeptic in me tightened my shackles.

I sat in a straight-back wooden chair against a wall in a dimly lit tiny office and he sat practically next to me, in front of his desk beside me. You've seen or heard the 'close your eyes' routine. And then in a softly soothing tone over a few minutes, he asked me to relax my legs, upper arms, down my arms to my hand, while he seemed to chit chat about other unimportant things. Finally he said my arm was totally relaxed. He said it was so light that it could rise from the armrest. The strange thing was that my arm actually felt heavy being so relaxed, but sure enough, my hand and arm left the chair, and dangled in midair. Hypnosis, or whatever, I don't want to keep you dangling, and I'll get to the punch line.

For quite some time, over a year or two, I could turn that on at will by myself. I did the same thing to my young teen children, and it had the same effect. Over the last few years, I didn't give it much thought. I didn't need it because my problem didn't have a hold on me so much anymore. So, I wasn't doing it. A month ago, I thought about that wonderful relaxation technique and wondered if I could still summon it at will. After producing the correct environment, it took me the same five minutes to get that deep, that quick. My brain had incorporated the technique like riding a bike.

So, there are multiple ways to mentally relax, some may fall under meditation techniques and some are also physical, like yoga. Find out what works for you in your transitional decade. It may be different than your earlier years. Perhaps ten years ago your first inclination was to use four letter words while ensnarled in Golden Gate Bridge traffic or the Long Island Expressway. But now, you're older and wiser, and instead, your mind is calm and collected as you listen to soft NPR music and realize you can go home and perhaps hypnotize your arm to dangle in mid-air if you so choose.

———

This book should highlight things you shouldn't do and the reasons why, but also reinforce positive actions. This is one of my favorites – it's called productivity. Productivity should create enthusiasm in your life. I also believe the opposite is true. The more enthusiastic you are, the more productive you will be. They also go hand in hand with kindling your *spirit*.

Do you ever notice a child when they have something to show you, something they just made? They run over to you, face aglow, construction paper flapping in their hands, and they practically jump into your lap. "Look what I made, look what I made," they may say. "Look at this Grandma," or Grandpa, or Mom or Dad, or whoever, as the case may be. The sense of pride of the picture they just drew and colored is immense. If you love your work and put in effort on a fine project, you also glow anew with a job well done. Be it an engineering project, an artist's creation, completion of a fine book, a business presentation, a doctor making a difficult diagnosis – the list goes on. It's what human beings have intuitively done for thousands of years, is to be productive. It's when we are handed things on a silver plate and/or learn to be lazy and non-productive that our spirits die.

To demonstrate how important productivity is and how that word packs such a powerful punch, I'll give you some synonyms for the word productive from a variety of sources. Roll them over in your head. They are so potent.

Advantageous, Beneficial, Constructive

Effective, Energetic, Fruitful

Gratifying, Helpful, Inventive

Producing, Profitable, Prolific

Rewarding, Rich, Teeming

Useful, Valuable,

Vigorous, and Worthwhile

I won't get into physical productivity or actual exercising in this chapter because we'll cover that big one later. Keep your mind active by maintaining problem solving skills, being artistically creative, and being productive with your job or career if you're still working. Do not sit back and get complacent. Do not get lazy. Do not watch television most of your day or surf the internet aimlessly to shop or chat. On the other hand, if you are too busy trying to fulfill obligations, cut back on them. Schedule and prepare your time more thoughtfully to be productive with things that are gratifying. Set a pattern for the transitional decade of smart time scheduling and preparation for activities that interest you, are rewarding, and make you more productive.

Do you like to knit or crochet? Do you want to learn about fishing? Do you do crossword puzzles? Have you ever taken up painting or the piano? Do you enjoy gardening?

You don't have to take piano lessons if your son's piano is still at home and you don't know how to play. You may purchase a piano book and at least teach yourself the basics of the black and white keys and surprise your spouse and yourself by learning the amateur, fun, and rewarding pieces in a beginner's booklet.

Why don't you plant a different group of plants that you haven't tried? Branch out to a small vegetable garden. The effort of planting tomatoes is well worth the rewards of the juicy, red beefsteaks you'll be slicing in the summer.

Is there a local school nearby teaching adult education courses? Look up a computer course if you need to modernize your knowledge of computers. Learn how to become a webmaster. Your kids won't believe it.

Do the daily newspaper's Sudoku and crossword puzzle. Filling in those boxes a bit more each week will make you feel smarter. Maybe you've never done them before so you feel intimidated, but if you live to 85, you'll be a whiz in another ten years and have many years left to be super smart with them.

I love this one. Start writing essays of your life's experiences or tackle the start of your memoir for your children and grandchildren. Yes, you can do it. Computers make the task so much easier.

Did I mention volunteer work? The possibilities are endless.

Chapter 6
How Is Your Body Changing?

Do you ever assume your spouse or child knows something when they don't? I am guilty of that a lot. On the other hand, when you tell a person something informative or factual, you have to be careful it doesn't come across as a lecture.

Since M.D.s go through significant amounts of training, and the day in and day out of a daily medical practice, sometimes we forget that lay people aren't aware of some of the basic information that we and other health care professionals possess. I'd like to share with you some physiologic changes, besides our lungs, that our bodies slide into during the transitional decade and beyond. Gaining this insight will help you better understand all the other aspects of the do's and don'ts in the other chapters.

Here's a common problem. You hear people use this term almost casually but not undeserved. It's dehydration. It's especially difficult on us as we age and I'm going to tell you why. Besides the elderly, it can happen to sport enthusiasts and especially to people in the summer who are less acclimatized to hot, humid weather. Like last summer, when a neighbor who isn't a regular golfer, played all day, and didn't keep up with the Gatorade quota for 18 holes.

Again, people who are busy with other careers have a varied understanding of dehydration and drinking fluids, but most don't know the underlying principles. Knowing more will be an asset, especially if the time ever comes when you experience the symptoms we'll talk about.

A certain percentage of your body weight is total body water. The amount of water is affected by your lean body mass, but it's also dependent on your age. Males and females differ because males have, overall, all things being equal, a slighter greater water percentage. So I'll streamline my example with just female numbers.

A fourteen year old female is approximately 57% water. When she hits the transitional decade she will be approximately 47% total body water and over sixty she'll be less than that, but not significantly.

I'll expand this simplification to say that our total body water is divided into two parts. If we are about 60% water, then about 40% will be fluid that is inside our cells and 20% is fluid that is outside our cells. What's going on with these different compartments and in the fluid, is the exchange and distribution of electrolytes – for instance – sodium, potassium and your main protein albumin.

So, we "older" folks have less body water than we did when we were younger.

Let's take a cursory look at the electrolytes I just mentioned. If you lose too much water without the sodium, the sodium is going to get concentrated, right? This is a common form of volume depletion. It's called hypernatremia (high sodium). Wow, can there be symptoms with that! Your nervous system doesn't like that very much. Concentrated sodium can cause lethargy, muscles problems, and even seizures. Shock can develop due to dehydration.

With the above example we looked at a shift in the electrolytes. Electrolytes are measured in blood work when you go to the doctor's office or hospital. When you see those bags of IV fluids hanging near a patient's bed in the hospital or during surgery, they have been picked to give the patient what he or she is low in, or they are picked to dilute solutes that may be too high, such as the high sodium in the above example.

Let's say you are in the transitional decade and you have a spirited tennis match in the heat after skipping breakfast. You don't bring a water bottle because you're thinking of hydrating and eating lunch out after the match. You finish with a loss, sit on the bench, and feel woozy when you stand up. Your heart rate seems to be a bit speedy and your mouth is dry.

You are showing symptoms of volume depletion. You're dehydrated. You may have played the same amount of time, in the same type of heat fifteen years earlier, but now you have symptoms quicker because you have aged and have less fluid flowing around your body to cushion against loss.

What if you're on the infamous diuretic, one of the first mainstream meds for high blood pressure? That will compound your dehydration status.

So, the bottom line is to drink plenty of fluids under normal circumstances and more so if you're physically exerting yourself, sweating, or running a fever.

Let's talk about kidneys and then I'll highlight a few more things.

What's the big deal with kidneys and aging? You may be sitting there saying you don't care, but your kidneys are important because what goes in must come out, or thereabouts. An average sized adult takes in two liters of water (or its equivalent) a day and excretes one and one-half liters of water. To give you some US equivalents, a gallon is roughly four liters, so we're talking about less than half a gallon of liquid in and out per day.

Your kidneys have the highest blood supply of all tissues. During the transitional decade we have less water volume. Our kidneys are receiving less flow; they are aging and have less mass, and their secretory and reabsorption abilities decline. You are more at risk again for dehydration. What is another consequence of our kidneys slowing down? The medications you are on may have increased bloodstream drug levels. If you become dehydrated, the concentration of several acetaminophens you took for pain increases, and your liver doesn't like concentrated Tylenol.

See how it works? One thing leads to another.

I've set the stage for you before we get to the next chapter on alcohol. You're going to be a whiz at understanding my points on alcohol.

———

How about other physiological changes? Have you noticed your height declining? I seem to have taken the plunge in the last two years and I don't like it. I've lost two inches. Where did it go? With loss of total body water, the tissues between the bones in your spine has less cushioning (like dried sponges), so those bones or vertebrae sink closer into each other. Also, you have less skeletal and muscle mass.

Sure, the bone mass is another problem. You are more apt to fall. And of course, our joints get tight so that we need some kind of WD-40. Besides osteoarthritis, Americans seem to be bombarded with television ads for products to prevent osteoporosis. I think the incidence of osteoporosis is going to take a giant leap and it already affects 55% of Americans over fifty-years old. Do you ever see a young person drinking milk anymore? I drank milk growing up but ditched it as an adult, and my bone density results teeter on osteopenia/osteoporosis. I shudder to consider the next generation's crumbling bones.

Don't forget about your eyes. Pupillary dilation and constriction takes more time. It goes along with what people say – how old people don't have the adequate reflexes to drive. It starts with their eyes, and then their body movements are slow, too. It's a real problem, so much so, that the young ones want to take Grandpa's license away from him. Wouldn't we all be safer?

If you're in your fifties, then it shouldn't be this bad. However, I know that oncoming car headlights at night on the surrounding country roads are already bothering me. Cataracts, or clouding of the lens in your eye, are practically synonymous with aging. You can get away with it for awhile, but sooner or later, you'll be in an outpatient preop stretcher waiting line to have them removed. There is no other way to get around it – have surgery or get blinded by them.

Please book me into a laboratory research bubble as a guinea pig and fix my telomeres, please. And by the way, I really recommend you see an eye doctor if you haven't done so in several years. An optometrist is okay once in awhile for a quick change of prescription glasses, but during the transitional decade you owe it to yourself to see an Ophthalmologist. An Ophthalmologist is an eye doctor who has gone to medical school and went through a specialized residency and is knowledgeable about diseases as well as eyes. He or she is also trained in eye surgeries.

Chapter 7
Alcohol

Don't skip this chapter just because you think you're not an alcoholic. There's good information here for all of us and it may identify the people who are in denial about their alcohol consumption. You are not sitting in a therapist's office, or a doctor's office, or with your significant other. It's just you and your book, so I want you to be honest with yourself. We're going to start off by having you consider the answers to the following questions. It's not a test but a time for reflection. Don't forget all the things we've talked about and how we must keep away the *disorders* which make our transitional decade aging process worse than it should be.

How often (daily, weekly, monthly) do you drink a beverage with alcohol?

How many drinks will you consume while you are drinking?

If you start, can you stop with one?

Do you have to follow your previous night's alcohol with alcohol in the morning?

Has a friend or loved one shown concern over your drinking?

Has drinking interfered with your work production or other activity?

Have you had a sneaky suspicion or a guilt that you've had too much?

If you are feeling uncomfortable because some of your answers may be incriminating – then perhaps you *are* drinking too much. Or perhaps you're still not sure. What constitutes a drink anyway? A couple of beers starting around lunch time doesn't really count, right? "All the guys have beer on the golf course," you say.

"There's nothing wrong with that." Except that these retired golfers play almost every day!

I rarely drink, but I have my favorites just like most people. Irish cream liqueur, Amaretto, a whiskey sour, or my favorite honey wildflower wine. But if I open a bottle of wine, it may still be in the refrigerator a month later if I don't have someone to share it with. And the liqueurs? It varies, but suffice to say, they last a long time.

It doesn't sound like much, but about 0.6 fluid ounces or 1.2 tablespoons of pure alcohol mixed in your beverage constitutes a drink. Here are more equivalents of an alcoholic drink:

A single shot glass (1.5 ounces) of alcohol such as 80-proof whiskey or gin (that's about 40% alcohol),

Five ounces of table wine (that's about 12% alcohol),

Twelve ounces of beer or a cooler - that is about 5% alcohol.

If you drink two twelve ounce beers, that's already two "drinks," and if you were to polish off a 750 ml bottle of wine, you've had five drinks. It adds up, doesn't it? The point is that what constitutes a drink is a lot less than the average person would admit.

Alcohol can do nasty things to your body. Your aging body's organ systems don't need to be aggravated any further. Alcohol can damage your brain, your liver, your pancreas, and other parts of your nervous system.

Have you heard of cirrhosis of the liver due to alcoholism? Alcohol breaks down in the liver; yet it starts to kill off the very cells needed to metabolize it. The liver is extremely important in metabolizing drugs and absorbing major nutrients such as vitamins A, D, E and K, proteins and fat. Alcohol disrupts that process. Aging in the transitional decade has already caused your liver to lose some of its mass. Less blood flows through its hepatocytes and it has less metabolic activity due to decreased enzymatic action. Don't compound the problem by drinking in excess.

Not that we are young party animals, but how come on TV or in the movies, more consistently than not, you see people at parties drinking and having a good time, hyped up happy? Alcohol is a downer. Really – it's a depressant. Particularly in the elderly, it can precipitate depression, not to mention the fact that it causes less inhibition. In addition, someone could get hurt if you get behind the wheel after drinking, even if you haven't reached the "legal limit." That could result in a serious disruption to the rest of your life – physically, mentally, and legally – as well as someone else's.

Alcohol is sinister in another way. It affects people differently. One drink for one person may be another person's level for intoxication. It also depends on your fluid status. We talked about volume status. If you are dehydrated, watch out. I know someone recently who did his after-work run of a few miles, missed dinner with his buddies, but caught up with them for a beer. Well, this healthy young person had two beers and a margarita, passed out, and was sent to the ER where he had to be, what? Rehydrated with IV fluids because he was dehydrated and to dilute the alcohol in his bloodstream.

Not only does alcohol have detrimental effects if you're dehydrated, but think of it as a diuretic. Don't you run to the restroom more often when you're drinking? So here we go again, another trigger of dehydration. Now we have a bigger mess.

The effects of alcohol consumption are also dependent on coexisting conditions you may have and the medications you're taking.

So is it worth it to have more than the occasional one or two drinks? Also, don't forget that alcoholism is a progressive disease and once you start "drinking," you're going to crave that margarita or scotch sour, beer or whiskey. And if you've let it go too far, the true alcoholic will have the most unpleasant symptoms when he tries to stop. How about terrible anxiety, hallucinations, even convulsions?

Cutting back on your alcohol consumption takes planning and guts. That kind of change is not easy, but you'll be surprised to see how many people will support you if you let them know. First, admit and keep track of how much you're drinking. If you don't need professional help, set your own goals, pace and decrease your normal consumption, eat before you drink, and avoid the situations that cause you to drink at all or too much. Don't give in when others want you to drink. This is about your liver and aging, not theirs. Do the right thing for you.

If you are drinking in excess and you need professional help, go get it. A physician can prescribe medications which can ease the pangs of withdrawal when trying to quit. He or she may also want blood drawn for comprehensive testing. You may need a specific diet or supplements to replace your B, A, D and E vitamins. In addition, there is always therapy and AA.

_____

What follows is the Alcohol Use Disorders Identification Test, or AUDIT test, which is well tested to be valid and reliable as a screening tool for alcoholism. I believe it is an extremely useful tool so please thoughtfully consider your answers and record your scores for each line. Again, no one is watching you, judging you, or going to give you a lecture. It's a serious questionnaire and the truthful score should give you something to think about. The highest score is 40.

Questions	0	1	2	3	4
1. How often do you have a drink containing alcohol?	Never	Monthly or less	2 to 4 times a month	2 to 3 times a week	4 or more times a week
2. How many drinks containing alcohol do you have on a typical day when you are drinking?	1 or 2	3 or 4	5 or 6	7 to 9	10 or more
3. How often do you have 5 or more drinks on one occasion?	Never	Less than monthly	Monthly	Weekly	Daily or almost daily
4. How often during the last year have you found that you were not able to stop drinking once you had started?	Never	Less than monthly	Monthly	Weekly	Daily or almost daily
5. How often during the last year have you failed to do what was normally expected of you because of drinking?	Never	Less than monthly	Monthly	Weekly	Daily or almost daily
6. How often during the last year have you needed a first drink in the morning to get yourself going after a heavy drinking session?	Never	Less than monthly	Monthly	Weekly	Daily or almost daily
7. How often during the last year have you had a feeling of guilt or remorse after drinking?	Never	Less than monthly	Monthly	Weekly	Daily or almost daily
8. How often during the last year have you been unable to remember what happened the night before because of your drinking?	Never	Less than monthly	Monthly	Weekly	Daily or almost daily
9. Have you or someone else been injured because of your drinking?	No		Yes, but not in the last year		Yes, during the last year
10. Has a relative, friend, doctor, or other health care worker been concerned about your drinking or suggested you cut down?	No		Yes, but not in the last year		Yes, during the last year
					Total

***

Positive screens for heavy drinking are:
For men up to 60 years old: total score of 8 or higher;
For women: a total score of 4 or more.

I hope this chapter was informative. You may have gained insight into a problem which you have averted, and others, I hope, will decrease their drinking habit or see their primary care physician for help in tackling their alcohol consumption. Or, please consider AA (Alcoholics Anonymous).

Chapter 8
Stress

Stress!

Over time, no one is exempt from this one.

You are in your fifties and you've handled the major moves, the child rearing, the ups and downs with careers, the loss of loved ones, the financial pitfalls. Some of these items may still be on your plate. Look, it's time to start diverting your problems, your anxiety, and your stress to the periphery of your life. With whatever time you still have left on this side of the ground, let's diminish your stress.

I believe there are two types of stress, neither of which are any good. The first type is the stress disorders. It is possible to have an acute stressful event several weeks after being subjected to a traumatic event. This is shorter lived than the other disorder called posttraumatic stress disorder, PTSD, which we hear so much about from men or women who return to civilian life after horrible wartime events. I will never forget, while rotating in psychiatry as a medical student, the Vietnam vet who stoically related his recurring memories of emotional trauma which precipitated his PTSD and depression. He came into a circular field where there were several soldiers' dead bodies with sacks over their heads tied with rope at their necks. He and his comrades undid the burlap sacks to find the rats which had been included, gnawing away at their faces. Imagine his horror and helplessness reliving that experience in his mind on a regular basis.

These two types of stress disorders are prime examples of how stress can impact us medically straight away into a diagnosis and medical treatment plan.

So what exactly is stress other than the disorders above? Do only type A personalities get it, and what are the symptoms?

Here's a helpful way to think of stress. Have you ever heard of a stress fracture? Think of a force or pressure which strains or deforms a bone. Now translate that physical stress to a mental pressure or tension. It can do some damage there, too, because then your brain is in overdrive and signals your adrenal gland to release hormones at higher than usual levels. Cortisol and adrenaline levels should usually be at normal, low, and steady blood levels.

It's okay for these flight or fright hormones to be released once in awhile if you lose your car keys, or if your cat knocks an item off your night stand in the middle of the night; but if you chronically have high levels in your bloodstream, your body is going to age more quickly in your transitional decade.

Think of adrenaline as the sprinter. It causes your heart to tick faster and your blood pressure to go higher. It may even come from having a white-coat syndrome while being checked into your doctor's office; you're worried over your appointment, and your blood pressure goes higher. You then have something to worry about when she walks in.

What about cortisol? When your mind is constantly under stress and pressure, the pituitary gland releases too much ACTH, a hormone, which causes your adrenal gland to increase its release of cortisol. I think of cortisol as adrenaline's counter balance. It tends to dampen your normal immune responses, digestive system and other functions while adrenaline is making you act like a sprinter. With this one example, you can see how you would be affected if the stress was turned on almost all the time. Your body's immune system, partially responsible for keeping you well and healthy, becomes weakened with too much cortisol.

Cortisol also causes glucose intolerance. The sugar which is stored in your body is broken down, increasing the level in your bloodstream. Think of another thing that is more common in our transitional decade, especially if you're putting on the pounds – Type II Diabetes, or non-insulin dependent diabetes. If you're living with too much stress, that's a double whammy to be increasing your blood sugars with a potential, or a full diagnosis of diabetes. We will, however, talk more about diabetes when I address the Disorders.

Not sleeping well at night? It could be due to all that stress. Do you have indigestion or ulcers, find yourself fatigued, have more headaches than before, or unexplained backaches? How is your memory these days? Do you know that all those beauty facial products won't do much if your stress manifests itself as a skin problem like eczema?

––––––

Stress doesn't discriminate. It doesn't seek out only the rich or the politicians, the skilled laborers or professionals, the unemployed or the Hollywood actors. It happens to all of us but here's the thing - we all handle our problems differently. Someone's crisis may be another man or woman's mere annoyance. So learning how to cope with stress is imperative. The more you learn to handle problems effectively as life goes along, the less stressed you will be as more serious ones come along.

You must develop techniques which work for you. There will be situations in your life which you cannot change and they are so taxing and draining that you wish you could run away. This is especially true if you taking care of a family member with Alzheimer's or a debilitating illness. That is when you must seek out a professional organization's help to support the caregiver. There are multiple examples of this scenario. Often the caregiver needs a large dose of mental encouragement and a day off to recoup his or her spirit. Do it, please.

Let's look at some useful ways to get unstressed. There's a difference here – it's not necessary to go back to the things we mentioned about being productive. If your mind is cluttered with persistent thoughts of the lousy dead-end job you have and the insolent behavior thrown at you from an arrogant boss, then you should focus on displacing your thoughts. You don't have to be productive, although that wouldn't be a bad thing.

You already know one of the remedies for just about anything – exercise. I'll devote a chapter to exercise, but here's the low-down for this scenario. Exercise is a good remedy for many things, but unless you take that two mile run, or that one mile swim, or that one hour on a treadmill, and *not* think about your stupid boss and how you got passed over for a raise when you do all the work, then you haven't tapered down your stress levels, have you?

In many instances, the key is controlling your thoughts. You have to channel your thoughts to prevent your brain from sending all those pituitary hormones down to your adrenal gland. I'm going to put on my thinking cap while you do the same. Let's think of a variety of activities where you must focus on that *one* thing – from sedentary to active.

Do you play chess? Learn how. If you're concentrating and playing to win, you're thinking about your next move. Same goes for card games.

Read a totally engrossing book.

Do you play an instrument? Take lessons – this will stimulate your creative genius and destress you at the same time.

If you don't know yoga and meditation, yet may be interested, find some credentialed instructors and go for it.

Schedule an occasional massage. This is so therapeutic - your body is thoroughly kneaded into putty...your mind can't help but follow.

Sports – if you play with an opponent, you'll have an active mental game. You don't know what the other player is going to do so your mind can't wander to your problems. Racquetball, tennis, and squash are good examples, especially if your partner is as good or better than you.

If you like to swim, but swim lap lanes at a slow or moderate pace, your thoughts may not be on your swimming. Varying your sets, strokes, and speed should help.

For golfers, they still have cart time or walking time between hitting that ball. But it's better than many other activities and often there are lively conversations and jokes being told between players. However, stress can ruin a golf game as scores are directly proportional to stress levels!

Make sure you are getting enough sleep. This is a double-edged sword. If you aren't rested enough, that may be causing you to more easily get stressed. And yet, if you are stressed already, that will prevent you from sleeping well. Try to set a regular night time routine. Don't overeat or drink - including alcohol - late in the evening. Have a warm shower or bath. Get to bed and read or meditate a half hour before you would like to sleep. Do not address your problems at bedtime.

Another thing – that big city traffic. Leave earlier for work to give yourself some extra time in case there's a tie-up, or go a different, longer route that isn't so stressful. Try audio books to keep your mind off stress. As you listen to the narrator you forget your problems.

Now here's one of my favorites - humor. Everyone has their own opinions about what's funny. Invest in buying what you consider to be the funniest DVDs, set aside the evening, and watch one. I bought my Dad the entire DVD set of *Mr. Bean* DVD comedy when he was mentally and physically failing, and for the last six months of his life he put them on all the time. I had never seen him laugh as much as he did in his last few months of life.

Have you seen *Rat Race*? You can throw some old classics in there, too, like *Some Like it Hot* with Marilyn Monroe, Jack Lemmon, and Tony Curtis. Go to a big box store online, search their DVDs, and you can find off-the-beaten path movies. They are worth the investment. And please, we're talking humor here – serious crimes and gunfire doesn't work.

We've talked enough about stress. Here's one more suggestion. Quantify your stress like we do in health care regarding pain scores. Take a piece of paper, draw columns from one to ten and put down days of the week. If you're going through a rough time, try the above suggestions, and every night over a month, score how your day went. Make ten the highest stressful score and try to see where you stand during the month, along with what measures you take to cope. You can then see if certain techniques work for you and others don't.

Good luck, beat your buddy at a game of chess, and enjoy those funny movies!

Chapter 9
Dogs

I give a talk on this subject. Are you aware of the big changes that have occurred in society regarding dogs?

First off, ponder these statistics from the Humane Society. In 2001, 36% of US households owned a dog and in 2008 that jumped to 39%. And something else interesting happened. The number of dogs in each household grew. Although 63% of those households owned one dog, 25% owned two dogs, and 12% owned three or more dogs. I give weight to the statistics. From 2001 to 2008, my husband and I became dog owners (after many, many years), then we also gained another dog, and then later, became a three dog-owner family.

There are baby boomers right now in the transitional decade. My suspicion is that they are responsible for the increase in dog ownership. As long as they don't take on more than they can handle, such as vet bills, boarding bills, lack of time, etc., then I think this is a step in the right direction as far as your health, well being, and spirit. Some people may come close to being your soul mate, close friend, or loving spouse, but there aren't going to be many people who love you as much as your dog. They don't care if you aren't wearing the newest fashion trend, live in a shack or a million dollar house, or if you've been laid off or were just promoted to VP of a major beer company. They love you because you're you.

———

Do you know that there is an airline devoted to pets, called "Pet Airways?" You can fly Fido like a paying passenger. Flights go from NY-Washington DC, Chicago, Denver to LA. Are you aware that some prime hotels have a resident dog in their lobbies so if you are missing your own Lassie while you're away on business, you can take the lobby dog for a walk or a run? The dogs are set up nicely with a bed, water, and sometimes a dog house. I have seen this in a four-star hotel across the river from MIT, and I've met Ben, a chocolate Lab, in a Sheraton Suites in Calgary, Canada.

Some college dorms have a new option. They are allowing dogs or other small pets less than 40 lbs. This may also happen in the future – a law for at least one resident pet to live in a care facility. There are also full semester college courses on animals in society, and the students must gain some personal experience in animal work therapy.

———

Dogs and cats are a fundamental part of our existence. They have been around a long time and have influenced past societies and medicine. We should know better than to disrupt their coexistence with us; after all, they have a genetic predisposition to hunt and protect and provide us with companionship.

In the 1300's, twenty-five million Europeans died in five years from the Black Plague. That was one-third of Europe's population. Superstition, witchcraft, and the church contributed to the mass murder of Europe's cats which caused the rat population to proliferate along with their fleas. The flea-borne infection with gram negative Yersinia Pestis caused the infamous Bubonic Plague. Some people prefer dogs over cats, but nevertheless, cats serve a purpose as well!

By the way, we own a cat, too. But she thinks she's one of the dogs.

———

You already know where I'm going with this – how important, in particular, a dog is to your well-being, especially in the transitional decade when you may have the empty nest syndrome. Dogs give unconditional love back to us which is good for our health and our spirit, and we're getting more factual with the data to help prove that, due to work with therapy dogs. So I'll fill you in on therapy dogs. Not only will you someday perhaps have a visit from a therapy dog and his or her handler, but you may want to consider training or getting a dog to train for therapy work. This will feed back into our productivity chapter. Dogs can be our best friends, are good for our spirit, health and productivity.

A therapy dog is not a service dog. A service dog assists his own owner whereas a therapy dog is handled by his owner to assist others at specific times. Here's another difference. Therapy dogs are not entitled to the same benefits that service dogs are. In essence, the Federal American Disabilities Act states that any dog assisting a person with a disability is considered a service dog and is entitled to freely access any building or form of transportation. A therapy dog does not have free access. His handler must ask permission for the same level of passage as a service dog.

Something else about a therapy dog is important. The large therapy dog organizations provide an insurance policy on certified dogs while they are working. My therapy dog, who works with both the old and the young, has a million dollar policy. Some institutions are lax with a policy of allowing non-credentialed dogs. They allow dog owners to bring their pets through their facility because the handler simply says he or she is a "therapy" dog, but they are not insured nor are they tested and credentialed. The dog can be good as gold, but what if there was a mishap that wasn't the dog's fault? In this litigious society, it's not wise for a facility to have an owner come through with one of these dogs. You can trust a credentialed dog - most likely he will exhibit dependable and safe behavior under unusual circumstances.

A therapy dog's mission is to enhance the quality of life for people in a variety of environments. They can also be part of a physical, social, emotional, and/or cognitive function treatment plan. Articles and research are lining up to corroborate the beneficial effects therapy and pet dogs have on people. I will list the names of some journals in the Appendix if you'd like to search for published articles about animals and their benefits.

There appear to be long-term cardiovascular benefits in pet owners over non-pet owners, such as increased one-year survival rates of post heart attack patients. After a lung transplant, patients with pets have a better quality of life score as measured by a hospital questionnaire. Pets have a calming effect on your blood pressure and heart rate. Qualitatively, therapy dogs make nursing home patients in dementia units more alert and more apt to smile and interact. I often see it with my own dog. A visit from him lights them up, and although usually quiet, they'll ask questions about the dog, even if they are the same ones. ("What's his name? How old is he? How long 'ya had him?) Most people exhibit the child-like pleasure while stroking a dog around his ears or sinking their hand along his back, especially if he has big brown eyes glowing at them with appreciation.

Also, I am big on substitutions. When something gets taken away from your life, such as a loved one, there's nothing better to ease your pain than having some type of replacement. Yes, it's not the same, but this will help you swim rather than sink. It's actually what happened to me and yes, I actually needed two dogs. In the transitional decade, if you get a pup, just think of the good forthcoming years you'll spend with that dog.

Getting back to dogs outside the home, society is flourishing with new situations that incorporate dogs. They are in prisons, classrooms, elderly patient facilities, psychotherapy and depression treatments, speech therapy, seizure detection, hospice, funeral homes, cancer detection, and search and rescue. Also, they are probably a benefit to our society's health care costs.

———

Many of you may already have a dog or cat. And for some of you it may be impossible to own one because of your hours at work, or because of where you live, or perhaps because of your own health. Or maybe you have nasty allergies. Maybe when some of these issues resolve, you'll consider becoming a pet owner.

Some of you, however, may be in the gray zone. I know a couple right now just like that. They enjoy dogs but never had one as a couple, and they've been married for forty years. Their long-distance son recently came to visit them with his one-year-old Akita. A mutual bond set in after only two days. The dog stood at their son's car when they were leaving and imploringly looked back at the couple as if, "Aren't you coming?" or "I'll miss you, too." This couple's excuse for not having a dog has been that they don't know how to care for one. Well, needless to say, I am an encouraging neighbor and I'm presently helping them find the perfect fit.

If your lifestyle can accommodate it, please consider getting a dog. If you already have one or more, you are already reaping the benefits. But you already know this.

Chapter 10
Sunshine and Spirit

Sunshine, sunlight, sunburns. Let's talk about the good, the bad, and the ugly regarding these topics. Yes, you know it - there are positive and negatives regarding sun exposure. Unfortunately, there's not much you can do about the damage that's already been done, but as with quitting smoking in the transitional decade, there are still benefits to be had by changing your habits right now.

Let's get the bad news over with first so that I leave this chapter on an optimistic note about the positive effects of sunshine. I hope, above all, that you weren't one of those young people who laid out on the beach, or roof, or backyard, unprotected, basking below that hot, fiery, yellow ball in the sky. And, yikes, with what you should know before my telling you, you certainly shouldn't still be doing it.

If you do the above, you are more likely to get sunburn, even with sunscreen. It's common to see first-degree sunburns on people at the beach. If a person's skin already looks red during the day, you can imagine how that's going to ripen by the evening. A second-degree sunburn not only causes skin reddening, it also leads to water blisters. You've just packed on more skin damage. With a third-degree burn, the skin will actually be oozing - a deeper layer of the skin has been charred, and more eruptions will occur. Your skin is the largest part of your body's integumentary system. It's purpose is to shield and protect your body. When it breaks down, it becomes a place for bacteria to grow and infections to proliferate. It's serious and needs medical attention. The other not so fun part of a third-degree burn is the pain you'll experience.

Those sensory receptors are going to be open to the air, screaming bloody murder at you.

Don't think that you won't get a burn if you are under a small beach umbrella or if you're in twenty-degree weather skiing. You can receive more ultraviolet rays due to reflections from snow, sand, water, or metal. And I always love this one because it ruined one of my vacations once when I was young. The first day I arrived at a beach resort it was cloudy. I put the sunscreen on but not methodically enough, and stayed out too long because it was so overcast. Sure enough, I found out by nightfall that I had toasted well done.

Sunscreen. Use it. Spread it on all exposed surfaces. My nephew visited us in Florida once and we spent a few hours on the beach. He applied sunscreen everywhere except the tops of his feet. What if your feet hurt so much that you can't put on your shoes? It wasn't good.

There is so much information out there anymore about sunscreens. Pick a double digit SPF, with UVA and UVB protection. UVA is the ultraviolet radiant which causes the long term effects like the leathery look and wrinkles. UVB will cause the lobster look. Choose the appropriate sunscreen for your activities such as one which is waterproof. Reapply it often because even an SPF 50 will need reapplication in a few hours. You can even wear SPF protection as a daily ritual. Every morning I apply a facial moisturizer with SPF 25. It's basic, I don't even think about it. But, I reapply or put sunscreen on if I'm out in the middle of the day without much shade.

Even better than sunscreen? Wear the appropriate clothing to prevent too much exposure. I wear a baseball cap or a wide brim straw hat outside year round except for the winter months. I wear mostly long sleeve shirts. There are lightweight long-sleeve cotton shirts and sun protective clothing. While boating or hopping in the water, I wear a UV swim shirt over my bathing suit. Unfortunately

I have found that with all my years of outdoor lap lane swimming I suffer the consequences of skin damage even though I religiously used sunscreen. So for me, the ultimate answer is to cover up.

Here's another biggie. UVA is not blocked by most windows. We have learned that for susceptible people, there's a difference in skin damage between their right and left arms. When you are driving, your left arm is exposed to greater quantities of sunlight than your right arm. This can cause sun damage to only your left arm. Here's my example: spots on my left arm have been dug out with a scalpel, frozen with liquid nitrogen, creamed with Aldara, and so forth from many years of long distance driving. Whereas, none of that has occurred with my right arm.

Here's a trick and one which needs to get more press. They do sell sun protectant sleeves. When I am driving wearing a short-sleeved top and getting sun exposure on the left, I pull up the blue sleeve I keep in my car. Presto. Sun exposure taken care of. I certainly don't want any more skin lesions.

Since many of us in the transitional decade are beginning to manifest skin problems, please let's minimize any further harmful sun exposure!

———

Now that we've touched on sunburns, exposure, and prevention, let's look more closely at other reactions to sunlight which manifest on our skin. I can't stress enough that in the transitional decade, previous sun worshippers may end up with the leathery look. Wrinkles will be more prevalent, as well as small, whitish areas which are actually from depigmentation. But, the worst scenario is cancer.

Actinic keratoses are small pink or grayish spots on skin which crust or get scaly. Although they can have irregular borders like a cancer lesion, they are considered precancerous. Always see a medical doctor or a dermatologist if you're unsure about skin problems. These lesions can be treated with topical treatments.

Basal cell carcinoma is quite common. It often shows up on the face, around the nose. It may look shiny at first but then it becomes more like an ulcer. Like I did for a short time, you may tend to dismiss it because the lesions come and go. But it's being sneaky. If you dismiss it, you may become a patient who needs extensive surgery because it's eating away alongside your nose! Definitely see a doctor. If you catch basal cell early enough, your chances of surgery diminish and you may be able to treat it with topical ointments.

Squamous cell carcinoma also likes the face and ears. It is also a skin disturbance which will ulcerate and not heal. If this goes on, a skin graft may be needed to fill the surgical skin removal.

Malignant melanoma is a cancer that starts deeper in the skin and is more ominous. Many people have heard of it, yet they need to be on the lookout for new mole-type skin lesions which may have irregular borders and are often heterogeneous with a brown or darker color. Melanoma is something to definitely watch out for in the transitional decade.

See your doctor or find a dermatologist if anything concerns you about your skin, especially on your arms, legs, or face; especially if it will not heal and you're a fair skinned blonde or red head. You may be in denial in front of the mirror if that spot on your body has lingered for some time or you keep picking at it to make it go away. If it looks angry, ulcerated, irregular, bleeds, crusts, and seems to be getting bigger, then see your doctor. The thing may not even hurt, but it's a problem.

———

Now that I've warned you about the dangers of too much sun exposure, I'll tell you what it's good for.

Have you heard of SAD? Aptly named, that stands for Seasonal Affective Disorder. If you haven't heard of it, you may find out why your exacerbated bout each winter of cabin fever with the "blues" may be more than that. It's a type of depression that occurs in more northern climates and is seen more frequently in females. If for two or more years you have depression during the winter which goes away during the summer, and it's not due to other specific reasons, then you may have SAD.

Depressive symptoms may be typical of a normal "depression" such as lack of energy, oversleeping, feeling hopeless, and losing interest in social encounters or activities. If your concentration diminishes, your work may suffer, or if you withdraw from loved ones, relationships may be compromised. You may resort to wanting those extra alcoholic beverages we spoke about in Chapter 7 or yearn to eat sugary foods addressed in Chapter 4.

During winter, the sunlight hours and intensity of light decrease which causes a decrease in a brain neurotransmitter called serotonin. The hormone melatonin, whose release increases in darkness, may also be involved.

For those of us in the transitional decade, SAD may be associated with age.

The first and most natural treatment of SAD is light and sunshine. Okay, it may not be beach weather, but open your blinds and your shades and your drapes. Quit hibernating in the semi-dark in front of the fireplace. Go out. Take a walk with your dog from Chapter 9, take a hike, or snow ski. But get out for light exposure. After all, you don't have to worry about a sunburn unless you're on a ski slope and now you know you should apply sunscreen and protect the middle of your face with goggles.

There are other treatments for SAD, including anti-depressants and supplements. See your doctor if you need an evaluation and possible prescription. Also, if you are faced with a bad bout of SAD and the fresh outdoor weather isn't cooperating, there is always psychotherapy or light therapy. Discuss this with your doctor and look into a light therapy box. A pharmacist can help as well.

So, see, sunlight does play a part in your *spirit.*

———

Do you know the other important reason to get light or sun exposure? We're going to talk about Vitamin D, especially for the transitional decade. Women are probably more familiar with this one because it's no secret that many American women are falling short on their bone density tests. By the time I'm finished, I hope you'll understand the reasons why some sunshine is important and plays a role with Vitamin D and calcium, both necessary for your health.

Up until November 2010, the Institute of Medicine in Washington suggested the RDA, or recommended daily allowance, of Vitamin D for men and women between the ages of nine and fifty was 200 IU. For those of us in our fifties up to age seventy, that amount doubled, and over seventy it went to 600 IU. But the tables have been revised. The RDA from age one to sixty-nine is now 600 IU and for over seventy, it's 800 IU. It's clear for those of us over fifty and into our senior years, we're leading the pack for higher requirements of our daily dose of D.

Introductions are in order. Meet Vitamin D2 and Vitamin D3. Vitamin D2 comes from plants, but D3 is another story. 7-dehydrocholesterol is produced in skin cells. This compound then converts to a previtamin D3 by exposure to sunlight. The liver and the kidneys make further changes and we end up with the hormonally active form of vitamin D. That is called calcitriol (1, 25 – dihydroxycholecalciferol) and it increases the uptake of calcium from our GI tract and decreases the kidney's excretion of calcium into our urine.

So, our main and most significant levels of Vitamin D happen when we are subjected to UVB sun rays on our arms and legs and face. Sunshine raises our Vitamin D levels! We can take supplements and eat certain foods like egg yolks and fish liver oils but this method gives us a higher boost. So a few times a week when you're walking the dog for ten minutes, give your arms and face a little break from the "cover-up" for some rays.

What happens again to this acquired Vitamin D and what's the big deal with D? For children, it's responsible for the development of teeth and normal growth. In the intestine, Vitamin D is responsible for increasing the absorption of calcium and phosphorous.

You know that calcium is needed for your bones. Luckily for us, our parents insisted we drink milk as we were growing up. I hate to think of the generations behind us. Milk doesn't seem to be as cool as drinking soft drinks. Nevertheless, we women still seem to be lacking our fair share of calcium and Vitamin D, hence the need for the sunshine and the supplements. The biggest losers are the elderly who are in long-term care facilities or stay in their houses all day. They are the ones slipping right into a hip fracture.

If you have a complete physical at your doctor's office, it's easy to check your Vitamin D levels and check on your calcium status in routine blood work.

So, don't forget to take your sunshine walks and your calcium with Vitamin D supplements. Some Vitamin D food sources are eggs, milk, oatmeal, salmon, tuna, and liver. My favorites are salmon, oatmeal, and yogurt. I'll take vanilla yogurt, thank you.

Chapter 11
Disorders

I mentioned that during the transitional decade what makes the biggest difference in our health and decline are *disorders*. They make us older than our time. We're going to discuss the biggest culprits and the ones we can do something about. The way we do that is to live a lifestyle which prevents their unwanted occurrence to begin with.

I agree. It isn't easy. This is hard work because we don't live in the jungle where we have to fend for our next meal and we don't live in a preindustrial society when cars didn't take us from point A for dinner to point B for a decadent desert. We live today when a few bucks will allow us to put a tasty treat in our mouths requiring no energy expenditure on our part. For a reasonable price we can eat a thick juicy burger or steak along with melted butter streaming off a baked potato, or tasty, hot salty French fries. To savor outrageous ice cream flavors, all we have to do is make a selection from a huge grocery store freezer, whip out a debit card, and grab a spoon and a bowl at home.

There are two types of Diabetes Mellitus. You don't want to wish juvenile Type I on anyone. We're going to discuss Type 2 because it's the one to watch for in the transitional decade. Guess why I went on the above rant about eating? One reason was because obesity is a major factor in Type 2 diabetes.

Insulin is produced by the pancreas, which is tucked into the upper abdominal cavity. In Type 2 diabetes, either the pancreas does not secrete enough insulin, or our peripheral tissues become resistant to the effects of insulin. Since insulin regulates our body's ability to handle glucose, our blood level remains elevated with diabetes, particularly after a meal.

These are the important facts about what prolonged high blood glucose or hyperglycemia can do to you. I think of it like a sci-fi plot where glucose molecules plug up your tiniest blood vessels and afflict big blood vessels as well. There are well-known details about how this happens. The process involves nasty end products and proteins and evil chemical pathways and inflammation, but I'll point out what's important and what you should remember.

You may know someone now or in the past who can't feel the bottom of their feet, or who had a toe amputated, or years ago had their leg taken off after severe diabetic complications. You may have heard of someone who went blind and all you know is that they have diabetes. Perhaps your parent's friend has renal failure, receives dialysis treatments, and is diabetic.

Yes, this is what diabetes can lead to: retinopathy, nephropathy, and neuropathy, or damage to the small vessels of your eyes, your kidneys, and your nerves. How awful!

What if you realize in your sixties, after you've gained two pounds a year beginning in your early fifties, and you've slacked off year after year getting meaningful activity or exercise, that your hands and feet tingle or sometimes feel numb? Perhaps you feel a burning or sharp stabbing pain in your toes? You've gone to bed and all of a sudden it feels as though someone is jabbing your feet with needles? What if you are eating at a restaurant and you realize you can't focus across the room and that you've been in denial about your failing eyesight for some time?

You make an appointment with a doctor, get a full physical, blood work, and testing for diabetes, and on your return visit, he or she gives you the dreaded diagnosis. You learn that diabetes is quite preventable but now you exhibit end organ damage which you can't totally reverse. Wouldn't you be extremely annoyed at yourself? Hindsight for all of us is easy, but you're on the path right now to change your lifestyle before you end up at that terrible point.

Prevent Type 2 diabetes – keep your weight down and get regular activity. Don't burn out your pancreas. Let your body have a normal glucose load and insulin secretion.

Besides the little blood vessels we talked about, there are the large ones as well. Big vessel disease, or macrovascular disease, is bad - really bad. That ticker in your chest is fed its nutrients and its blood supply via big vessels, so if they end up clogged (atherosclerosis) then you can have chest pain (angina) or a heart attack (MI). I'm simplifying the situation and leaving out all that pathogenesis and cellular physiology because I'm getting from point A when you can prevent diabetes to point B when you've done all the wrong things and acquired it. I'm trying to scare you! If no one else will, I'll be the bad guy and put on the hat.

This is very important as well. Remember we said that as we get older we're more apt to get an infection than when we're younger? You'll have a double whammy with diabetes. Bacterial and fungal infections are more common. Women will be pestered with yeast infections and both genders will be bothered by foot infections. When you add the neuropathy and the loss of sensation, then the infections turn into ulcers, or worse.

So, please, before you get diabetes, don't overeat, get plenty of exercise (that Chapter is coming), limit your refined carbohydrates and increase dietary fiber. Go back to Chapter 4 for a refresher and eat lots of fruits and vegetables. Here's another trick besides the advice that you shouldn't grocery shop when you're hungry. At the supermarket before you check out with the cashier, evaluate what's in your basket. Did you stick that thick velvet cake with the gooey icing in your cart at the last minute? Remove it. Did you throw in a bag of assorted European wafer cookies or a container of malted milk balls? Take them out! From now on, the grocery store checkout counter is your appraisal time for making last minute sound eating decisions.

———

Are you ready for disorder number two? Just because many of your friends, or relatives, or one or both parents have this, it doesn't make it more acceptable to acquire. The topic is high blood pressure or hypertension.

This discussion slides right into our age bracket. Once we hit our fifties, our risk of getting high blood pressure increases. And did you know that more than half of us will have it by the time we're sixty-five?

As we get older, our arterial blood vessels transporting blood away from our pumping hearts get stiffer, which increases the resistance to blood flow. Think of blood pressure (BP) as pure math or physics. We learn in medical school that blood pressure equals cardiac output (volume of blood pumped by the heart per minute) times peripheral vascular resistance. So you see, if either of these increase, the blood pressure increases. "Resistance" is a key element.

You might also compare blood pressure to plumbing. High pressure damages pipes and similarly damages arteries. We can't escape aging and its adaptive changes in our blood vessels; so again, we must take steps to minimize the negative possibilities.

If you are in the transitional decade, you owe it to yourself, even if you have normal blood pressure, to sit down in the drug store or pharmacy section of your big box store and use the automated blood pressure machine once a week, or every other week. It is not enough to only get your blood pressure checked every few months or once a year at a doctor's office. And better yet, and I highly suggest this – buy your own blood pressure monitor called a sphymomanometer from the drug store. So here is my rule for this topic - buy your own BP machine. You'll have it for years, and you'll be monitoring yourself frequently at home the way you should be.

Although these machines are not always accurate, you will still gain insight by comparing your BP week by week. You'll know if those numbers are creeping up over time and not going back down. So what are those numbers? Patients and friends have asked me what those numbers mean. You know the arm cuff inflates and the reading is in mm Hg (millimeters of mercury). The top, higher number is the systolic pressure and the lower, bottom number is the diastolic pressure. The systolic is higher because it's the pressure in your arteries when your heart is pumping and when your heart then relaxes between beats, that's the diastolic measurement.

A blood pressure less than 120/80 is normal. Anything between that and 139/89 is considered prehypertension. Above 140/90 are the different stages of actual hypertension. You can also have isolated systolic hypertension and isolated diastolic hypertension. You know that hypertension can lead to a heart attack, other heart problems, or a stroke. But not only can hypertension cause health problems but other health problems, such as kidney disease, can also cause hypertension.

So doesn't it make sense to be checking your blood pressure routinely? Not only do you brush your teeth every day, but then you throw in flossing for a better clean up once in awhile, right? Or you may be using a special exfoliant or facial treatment once a week, or you color dab your roots once a month or get a haircut.

So don't you think you should be checking these two vital numbers regularly and watching any trends? Not checking these could result in a major health problem. Don't you think that's more important than worrying about your facial tone or hair color? Unlike many other health problems, hypertension can go undetected for a long time and you may not have any symptoms at all. Just think how hypertension can negatively affect your lifestyle if it causes heart problems or a devastating stroke.

There are folks who may be more susceptible to hypertension as well. Males have it more commonly at a younger age than females, and black people as well as those with a family history are at a greater risk. And along the lines of what we've been talking about, obesity, tobacco use, little exercise, and too much alcohol and stress will also increase those numbers you're monitoring. And if you've heard that too much salt at the dinner table isn't good for you, here's the reason. It contributes to hypertension because it's a fluid retainer.

It's apparent how our lifestyle choices all come together to make us healthy or not. We've laid out the basics. Here are the manageable things we can do to prevent hypertension:
- Follow Chapter 3's advice about not smoking
- Follow Chapter 4 about diet and weight
- Follow Chapter 7 about alcohol
- Follow Chapter 8 about stress
- Follow Chapter 11 about exercise

And besides monitoring your salt intake, you can look up a diet called DASH, the Dietary Approaches to Stop Hypertension, and implement what you can from Chapters 2, 5, 6, 9, 10, 12. And 13 may pay off, too.

What if despite your best attempts, your blood pressure slides upward and your doctor diagnosis hypertension?

I have heard this common complaint in the past from patients and loved ones: "I'm on too many blood pressure pills. I only want one."

In the short time during an office visit, it's difficult for a physician to take the time to explain the pharmacology of blood pressure medicine and all the data which supports it. It gets complex in any case, so it's not something you are apt to remember. I'll try my best to explain as simply as possible.

Probably everyone reading this knows what synergy means. I like to think of it like this. Let's say your two favorite ice cream flavors are vanilla and chocolate. On Monday, you have an ice cream cone with a double scoop of vanilla on a plain waffle cone, and it's quite good. On Tuesday, you have an ice cream cone with a double scoop of chocolate on a plain waffle cone, and it's also quite good. But on Wednesday, you have a scoop of vanilla and a scoop of chocolate on a plain waffle cone, which you find more satisfying than either two scoops of chocolate or two scoops of vanilla. It soars your spirits higher because it's as if your two favorite flavors are also on a chocolate-dipped waffle cone.

That's synergy, or the ability of a group to outperform its best individual members as Wikipedia would say. This is one reason your doctor may have you on two blood pressure medicines instead of one, especially if the first one wasn't doing the trick.

The number of available blood pressure medicines just keeps escalating. There are many classes or types of antihypertensives and then many drugs in each class. The different classes are unique from each other because of their mechanism of action. Then again, the medications in each class vary from each other in some pharmacologic way. These points are extremely important; your doctor chooses your antihypertensive for a specific reason. Usually, the first antihypertensive to be chosen is a water pill or thiazide diuretic which makes the restroom one of your best friends due to your kidneys working overtime to eliminate salt and water. It may moderate your blood pressure somewhat, but if the target pressure isn't met, your doctor may either increase the dose, or he or she may add another class to utilize another pathway to lower your pressure.

These are some of the more common classes of other medications which work on your heart, on your blood vessels, or on natural chemical pathways:

ACE inhibitors (angiotensin-converting enzyme inhibitors)

Angiotensin II receptor blockers
Beta blockers
Calcium channel blockers
Renin inhibitors
Vasodilators

Be sure to work with your doctor regarding your treatment goal, take your medication as instructed, and try your hardest to incorporate a healthy lifestyle, which brings me to my next topic under Disorders.

––––––

I must include the topic of cholesterol. You can easily get measurements of your lipid profile at your doctor's office, or some health fairs. If you don't see your doctor regularly, don't wait to see him or her every two years. Why don't you make an appointment once or twice a year and have your lipoprotein profile checked? Don't let your blood levels get unhealthy. You can't do something about unhealthy levels if you don't know they exist.

Perhaps I can help you understand your cholesterol numbers. Doesn't everyone get confused with what should be low and what should be high? There is HDL (high density lipoprotein) and LDL (low density lipoprotein) cholesterol. Are you healthier having the HDL high or low? Likewise, are you healthier having the LDL low or high?

You want your high density lipoprotein blood values to be high and your low density lipoprotein blood values to be low to have healthy lipid levels. It's best to keep LDL under 100 mg/dl and HDL higher than 60 mg/dl. When your LDL level goes above 100 and approaches 200 or above, your risk of atherogenesis and cardiovascular disease goes up. Atherogenesis means your arterial walls thicken due to fatty deposits. And cardiovascular disease is the leading cause of death in the United States.

Other values that are measured are total cholesterol and triglycerides. Almost one-hundred million adult Americans have a total blood cholesterol of 200 mg/dl or higher according to the National Heart, Lung, and Blood Institute. But, for total cholesterol, the desired value is less than 200! Triglycerides are another form of fat in your blood and that laboratory value is best kept under 150. If it goes higher than 200, risk becomes high.

We mentioned above that higher HDL levels are healthier. Does that mean if we independently raise them without changing other lipid parameters, we'll reduce our cardiovascular risk? No, we have to change other lipid parameters as well to make an overall healthy lipoprotein pattern. For such important and easily obtainable lab work, isn't getting your blood drawn worth it for the early diagnosis of abnormal lipoprotein values and subsequent modification of cardiovascular risk?

Lifestyle changes to help remedy risky lipid profiles are a primary strategy. How about following the suggestions we talked about with diet, weight reduction, smoking cessation, and what's coming later - exercise. Besides these chapters, you can find lots of encouragement from other books, nutritionists, exercise gurus, and your family physician.

As far as pharmacotherapy, you probably know someone on a statin. They are commonly prescribed to manage dyslipidemias and they specifically lower LDL levels. There are also agents to raise HDL, such as niacin or nicotinic acid, fish oils and fibrates. Niacin or Vitamin B3 has been shown to be very effective.

Here's the bottom line. Find out where you stand with a lipoprotein profile and don't be shy to ask your doctor to order one if you are in the transitional decade and haven't had one in several years. Tell him or her that your book doctor sent you and blame it on me!

Chapter 12
Caffeine and Sleep

Caffeine is touted as a cure all or a menace when it comes to several health issues. I want to touch on a few things, especially since we're going to talk about sleep.

We ingest caffeine from more than coffee and tea. It comes from cocoa beans, kola nuts, energy drinks, chocolate, diet pills, cold medications, and some pain relievers.

If you get a healthy dose of caffeine, your body may be so accustomed to it that your get a headache or irritable if you miss it for a day or two. So it is a tad addictive.

Caffeine gets metabolized through your liver. If you have caffeine in the morning, most of it will be gone by nighttime. It's advisable to curb your intake later in the day because it may affect your sleep. Besides the fact that it is a stimulant and causes nervousness, it depends on your sensitivity and caffeine history.

Did you know that if you consume too much caffeine, you could be spilling calcium and magnesium into your urine? We've talked about calcium and bones already. As you age, you know you need to hold on to what you get because of bone loss and weakening, especially with women. Let's not talk about adding milk to your coffee to balance out the possible calcium loss – let's try to limit the problem to begin with. This is reason number one why I have switched all my coffee use to decaffeinated. Yes, there is still some caffeine in it but I've taken a step in the right direction and yes, I also don't have any after the morning. And interestingly enough, my bone density test has concurrently stopped plummeting with further bad news.

Here's another caffeine subject, especially if you're female. Besides what I was formerly told or believed, I had a difficult time finding the correct information, studies, or literature on it, which confirmed to me that the medical jury is still out on who and what to believe.

Have you heard of a link between caffeine and fibrocystic disease? Over the years I have heard this correlation, even from a treating physician. However, search as I may, it does not appear in any of my medical textbooks. Benign breast lumps are related to hormonal changes, especially when a woman is premenstrual. Ouch, they can be tender and painful.

So, if caffeine does increase estrogen levels, then you could stretch things a bit to say that caffeine can add to a woman's lumpy breast problem. So, this is reason number two why I have switched to decaf. It can only help. As a matter of fact, since switching, I have had less needle aspirations and biopsies because of suspicious breast lumps.

I'll take only one more cup of decaf, thank you, and only in the morning.

What about our hearts and caffeine? Especially if you are not a regular coffee drinker, caffeine can affect your heart rate. You may already have an arrhythmia like atrial fibrillation, so don't you think laying off the coffee or drinking decaf in moderation, would be wise?

Getting a good night's sleep; don't we all love it? During our busy productive work years, we were often scurrying around trying to manage our time to get a full night's sleep. Now that we're in the transitional decade, maybe working less, retired, or working with the children launched on their own, we should theoretically have an easier schedule to get a full night's sleep. But, wouldn't you know it, as we age, one of our sleep stages gets shorter.

Sleep consumes so much of our lives, yet we hardly talk about it. Do you ever laugh at your dog, woofing and jerking his legs while deep asleep? Maybe he's off catching chipmunks, or eating a filet mignon, or following your footsteps on a long walk. Wouldn't it be nice to watch some of the fantastic excursions, people, places, and things we encounter in our dreams? It's another world when we doze off deeper and deeper into our REM stages each night. Our dreams take us into another reality. Why don't we do more research on tapping into this strange time away from our reality based lives? Anyway, I digress.

So what interferes with a good night's sleep, and what will enhance it?

Look back on your daytime activities if you're having trouble sleeping one or more nights in a row. Did you keep your coffee consumption to the morning? Did you sabotage yourself with a nap that was basically too long thereby taking too much of an edge off your tiredness to sleep at night? Were you a slug or a couch potato all day, or did you work at a desk, and didn't take a good walk to dissipate any energy? Did you not exercise in the past few days? Or did you get all your physical activity too close to bedtime, making you too invigorated?

However, this is a touchy topic. You may be on medications that cause insomnia, or you have medical problems that cause poor sleep. And if you're on pain medications or sleep aides, make sure you take them well ahead of bedtime.

Sticking to a dependable bedtime routine that works for you is important. Since my husband and I live in the woods and sleep early and rise early, our dogs are used to that. So when we are rarely up watching TV or a movie, and it turns 9:30 p.m., our Chesapeake Bay Retriever will stand off to the side, look back and forth to the adjacent bedroom, and woof at us. He will make his objections known and make us stick to the household schedule of locking up, lights out, and head to the bedroom. Nothing like a dog who's head of the household, and unbeknownst to him, looking after our health as well!

In city areas or facility living, the outside may be well lit for security reasons. I am used to sleeping in a very dark environment which only gets as light as the brightness of a full moon in the woods. For an extended time this year, I stayed at my Mom's assisted living facility where parking lot lights and path lights shone straight through light curtains and blinds. I slept well every night only after trying a comfortable sleep mask. And for noisy places, ear plugs are a must. Many people who work odd hours or shifts rely on them for sleeping during the day.

Here's another suggestion. When was the last time you bought yourself a fresh, fluffy pillow or a high cotton thread pillowcase? How heavenly comfortable! Go for it. You're in the transitional decade and you owe it to yourself.

You many fall asleep fine but perhaps you wake up restless in the middle of the night. Don't drink too much late in the evening, alcohol or otherwise. A stretched bladder wall will cause you to awaken because it wants to be relieved.

Okay, good night for now. It's time for bed before Chester starts barking at me and before we start working out with our exercise chapter tomorrow.

Chapter 13
Exercise

Some of you may be reading this book while pedaling on a bike at the gym. So, congrats on that, and I hope you worked up a vigorous and sweaty ride!

I saved the best for last. It ties into everything we've been talking about, including the ability to kindle your *spirit.* You'll see.

Have you ever mulled over this strange word exercise? I'd make a bet that it's one of the most common everyday words in our vocabulary, regardless if we are doing what it means. The word seems to have sprouted in language in the 14th century. I searched for this English word in an 1828 Noah Webster's dictionary and compared it to a modern dictionary to find no real difference.

However, this is what surprised me. The most common, modern meaning of exercise is the third or fourth definition down in order of priority. Before the meaning of bodily exertion important for health, comes the necessary movements (exercise of) or practice of your profession or work, and your practice (exercise of) religion, and the use of your senses or power of your mind or body (exercise your mind or eyesight).

Physical exercise is essential. Doesn't the word exercise need an overhaul to be slightly changed or given top billing? The physical activity/exertion definition of exercise should be number one in the dictionary. After all, in the 20th century, isn't this the first and main use of this word? Although we're using it so often, a great deal of our population isn't practicing it, which is one factor for the obesity problem discussed in Chapter 4.

Any active bodily movement we do that maintains or improves our health and fitness is exercise. We help our circulatory system, our heart, our muscles, maintenance of our weight, our immune system, our mood, and even our self esteem and athletic skills by exercising. We ward off obesity and the disorders we talked about and improve our sleep by exercising. We kindle our spirit and enjoy life so much more.

———

Since *Younger Next Decade* is geared towards those of us over fifty, I'm going to start with the sometimes forgotten topic of balance. It is important to work on your balance and coordination as you get older. Don't forget that balance and coordination decline as we get older and that clumsiness, and unsteadiness increases.

Beneath your brain's two cerebral hemispheres is a separate region called the cerebellum. Think of it as a fist tucked posteriorly beneath the hemispheres. Your spinal cord and areas of the cerebral hemispheres send the cerebellum sensory input which it then integrates. It is like a fine tuning control panel and enhances your motor activity to be more specific, accurate, and coordinated.

Granted, some of us are more comical than others with our motor skills. Chevy Chase gave meaning to falling. And yet others give motor coordination inhuman possibilities and stupendous appearances such as the French wire walker (*Man on Wire*) who stealthily crossed over from the top of one World Trade Tower to the other. Here's my point – Philippe Petit may have been genetically blessed, but with practice (and lots of it), he obtained incredible balance and coordination. At the end of *Man on Wire,* we see an older Philippe still working his fine-tuned skills.

Here's the point: use it or lose it. Your cerebellum needs to keep running smoothly, by sensory input, so that you remain balanced and coordinated. Another important component of balance is your inner ears. There is complex circuitry in your ears which interacts with your brain to coordinate your body's positioning and movements.

During any exercise routine, you should specifically incorporate exercises for balance. By doing so, you can keep or improve good balance, warding off falls and injuries. You may even be taking medications that disrupt proper balance. Exercising for balance is as simple as standing on one leg at a time for up to half a minute or so, or working up to it day-by-day. Even hiking or walking on uneven ground or paths can keep you mentally alert and focused on coordination. Ask an instructor at a gym, or get some manuals, or look up exercises for balance on the internet. I just checked, you can find some there. There's no excuse not to do this.

Before a word about gyms, I want to tie a short blurb right in here; something that seems to occur more and more as people get older. Clutter. Yes, clutter. It doesn't matter how much balance you hold onto, if you're a pack rat, and have magazine racks, standing lamps, ottomans, statues, large flower pots, and so forth, dotting your living quarters; you live in an obstacle course. All it takes is getting up to answer the phone in a hurry and tripping over something. You could end up with a lifestyle-altering injury. Was that debatable nice-looking ceramic vase with the plastic flowers worth it, *even if* a loved one gave it to you? If you hold onto it, put it up, alone, and out of the way.

Now, speaking of gyms. Do you know America's most user-friendly, accessible, and cost conscious gym-type facility for all family members? You're right: the YMCA. Look one up in your phone book. There are all ages, activities, and classes there. The traditional decade folks are blessed, because places like the Y offer off-hour activities when the kids and parents aren't so numerous, like water aerobics and yoga. And you'll find gym coaches ready to give you lessons. And yes, ask about specifics for balance and coordination.

———

Now we'll move forward to anaerobic, weight bearing exercise, but not without a word of warning. If you haven't been exercising for quite some time, and especially if you have some disorders already, including smoking or obesity, then see your doctor before beginning an active program to get in shape. You should know your blood pressure, too. Of course, you've already bought your sphygmomanometer.

Previously, I stressed exercises to improve your balance. Along with this, and as significant, is the role of strengthening your muscles and maintaining flexibility. You can't stand on one leg or do balance training if the muscles around your joints aren't strengthened. If you take a longer look at the older Philippe Petit's physique, you'll recognize he looks solid as a rock, his muscles are toned, and he exemplifies balance, coordination, flexibility, and strength which also must come from weight training. And by stretching, you train your muscles and joints to remain flexible with a good range of motion.

If you take on weight training, it's a good idea to pair up with an instructor or a class, at least in the beginning. What you learn can easily be incorporated into a household routine if you buy a small set of weights. You can also use a pound or two while you walk. (A suggestion for free weights is to recycle plastic milk containers filled with varying amounts of water). Using weights makes your muscles forcefully contract against a load. Not only will you gain strength, endurance and functional ability, but your heart will like it too. At the gym, you can use machines with weights. Mind you, we aren't talking about Arnold Schwartzeneger work outs here.

Do you know the difference between anaerobic exercise/weight training compared to aerobic exercise? It has to do with oxygen and biochemistry. Anaerobic actually means "without oxygen." Here, your muscles don't need oxygen, which tissues usually use, but your muscles get their power from glucose derived from glycogen which is broken down in the liver. Of course, here is where a healthy diet is also important. You won't have sufficient glycogen stored unless you're eating decent food with amino acids and carbohydrates from whole grains.

Also, the reason you won't need oxygen here on a biochemical level (of course, your body is still requiring oxygen and you are breathing), is because these activities are of short duration but intense, and do not only include weight training.

So fight back against the tendency of your muscles to atrophy as you age, and do some anaerobic exercising. And here's another pearl – your bones strengthen as well, which thwarts that dreaded osteoporosis. What a deal!

———

You already know that aerobic exercise is all about oxygen. You kick into aerobic metabolism if you exercise longer than a few minutes and get your heart rate up. Biochemically, you use oxygen to burn glucose and fat to form ATP, adenosine triphosphate, which is used for energy in all cells.

We said it's a good idea to see your doctor before a new exercise routine, especially if you are going to take up new or improved aerobic exercising. This includes bike riding, heavy hiking or climbing, swimming, cross country skiing, paddling a kayak, a racquet sport, etc.

Look at the benefits of aerobic exercise. It decreases your chances of morbidity, mortality, and getting one of those *disorders.* You can prevent cardiovascular disease! While exercising, your heart pumps a greater volume of blood, you increase oxygen uptake by tissues, and over time, you'll improve your baseline heart rate by slowing it down.

Getting into a reputable program or with a good instructor will help you get started. You need to determine the proper amount of activity. It's a balancing act because you want your body to have improved function but not at the expense of an injury.

Developing an exercise strategy should also incorporate a warm-up period and a cool down period before and after your aerobic exercise. Don't cut corners. Taking the time to do this can prevent injuries and warm up your muscles so you actually perform better. You should warm up with activities that are not stressful or fast, so you slowly ease into your real workout. Stretch your hamstrings, walk slowly, and then slowly begin your activity.

For example, start your stationary bike workout by stretching. Then, put the first five minutes on a low resistance; don't sweat, let your muscles warm up, and your circulation start bathing those hamstrings. Then move on to a better speed and resistance. If you are a real beginner, maybe it'll be best to have a 5 minute warm up, 10 minute more difficult ride, and 5 minutes to cool down. Increase that middle portion over time and your body will thank you for it.

Warming up by doing the activity you've set out to do is probably the easiest. After stretching at poolside, swim a few laps to warm up, and then get into your real swim. If you do an aquatics class, the instructor should give you adequate slower-paced activities to begin. And cooling down? It's basically the same concept as the warm up, but placed after your main cardiovascular workout.

———

Here's a good outline for what you should be doing if you are in reasonably good health and don't need specific precautions due to a *disorder.* (Although your doctor who takes your history and physical exam has the first say).

These are outstanding recommendations from the United States CDC (*2008 Physical Activity Guidelines for Americans)* on how much exercise you should be getting. It includes adults over 18 years of age, so this includes the transitional age and beyond. Sure enough, it includes both aerobic and anaerobic exercise which includes work on large muscle groups such as your legs, arms, back, hips, abdomen, chest, and shoulders.

Every **week**, you should do one of the following routines:

Moderately intense aerobic activity such as a fast walk: 2 ½ hours; and muscle strengthening activity - specifically work major muscles 2 or more days a week.

Vigorous intensity aerobic activity such as a run: 1 ¼ hours; and muscle strengthening activity - specifically work major muscles 2 or more days a week.

Aerobic activity which equivalently mixes moderate and vigorous intensity exercise; and muscle strengthening activity which works the major muscles 2 or more days a week.

If you can or are able, you should be following the above. But guess what? Better yet, you can do more. More is better. How about 5 hours of moderate intensity activity each week and you'll reap the reward with better health results? Yes, your time is limited, but this is worth it so try to increase any previous activity or take on the new ones above.

Consider this new information published in September 2011 from a study supported by the National Institutes of Health and published in the American Journal of Preventive Medicine which states that women who diet *and* exercise are more apt to prevent getting Type 2 diabetes. If women watching diet restrictions added on exercise, there seemed to be an added effect. Diet and exercise go hand in hand.

———

I have a few more things to say about exercise. Physical activity and all those good hormones escaping into your bloodstream lead to more *spirit*. Let's wrap up by naming the next chapter Exercise and Spirit.

Chapter 14
Exercise and Spirit

We can talk about diet, health, and exercise all we want, but let's attain the crème de la crème for the transitional decade and beyond. Bringing together the subjects we talked about, as much as possible, would be our ultimate goal. Practicing as many of them together can lead to what I believe is a joyous *spirit.* I'll share my own example.

Twice a week, by 7:30 a.m., I drive eleven miles to a hiking trail. Yes, it's early. I am afforded that luxury because my schedule is how I map it out. I am also a morning person, but nature is also glorious at that time. There's one more thing. If I wait until later in the day, other distractions may occur which prevent me from going, or I could possibly get too lazy. So I set off as soon as possible to make sure I get my exercise.

Remember Chapter 9? Of course, my buddy, my dog Chester, is with me. We're bonded. I'll have the luxury of carrying the leash without hooking him up, because he'll stay with me. I'm his main concern besides all the great smells he'll encounter. He's so excited to get on the trail, his tail never stops swooshing back and forth. His pleasure adds to my *spirit.*

The trail is in the woods along an embankment, some areas quite steep. It follows a river with three waterfalls, gloriously laid out so you pass the smallest first, the middle falls next, and after a twenty minute fast hike, you come to one that's over one-hundred feet. You can't take your eyes off the terrain, there are large tree roots and many areas with steps built into the dirt. At the end there are eighty steep metal steps. This is paradise for a hiker because you have to maintain balance and coordination on a constantly changing surface. It's a super cardiovascular hike with all the steps. I run up and down the areas with the most steps five times, for a total of approximately eight-hundred steps.

It's outdoors, and even though most of the trail is shady, I'm getting exposed to light for Vitamin D synthesis. Also, the air is magnificent. For a long time, I believed the air, especially around the big falls, was practically magical. While breathing there, I inhale the most fresh and purifying air I have ever encountered, especially when the water volume is at its highest in the spring, or after several days of heavy rainfall. It was here where I began believing in the theory about negative ions. They are molecules that have gained or lost an electrical charge. You breathe them in certain environments, such as around large waterfalls. When they are absorbed into our bloodstream, they may increase serotonin, which is a feel good chemical acting like an anti-depressant and stress reliever. In other words, a *spirit* enhancer.

I found this hiking trail and have incorporated it into my lifestyle. Look at all the things I accomplish with it, especially a cardiovascular workout which burns calories!

I didn't always use this activity – it was a substitution for something else. I used to be a huge swimmer. Then, I made sure that where I lived, I had access to indoor and outdoor lap pools. When a shoulder disability caused me to lose adequate range of motion, I could no longer swim, the thing I most loved to do. Rather than throw in the towel, my goal then was to find a substitute that I could be passionate about and incorporate the things I've been discussing.

You may be aware of people who don't have an entire limb, yet many of them go out and work the rest of their bodies to the max at the things they are passionate about. Isn't that the *spirit?*

———

Perhaps you like to have company when you exercise. You can start a walking program and invite a friend, or join a group at the YMCA. Even better, join a hiking club so you can walk challenging trails with other people like the one I mentioned.

Why not find a local river? If you don't have your own little paddle boat, many rivers have outdoorsman businesses nearby where you can rent a canoe or kayak. They'll get you launched, and they'll pick you back up in an hour downstream. The ones around here are reasonably priced, as well. But do you know that you can buy an inflatable kayak? It folds up and fits into a large canvas bag. You just throw it in your car with the paddle, air inflator, and life jacket, and bingo, you're off.

Also, just because you go on vacation or are on the road, doesn't mean you skip taking care of yourself. Besides making use of the hotel's gym, here's my favorite. It may not have a waterfall next to it, but it keeps me from being sedentary while away from my normal routine. I go to the hotel's stairwell and run or walk quickly, up and down the stairs. I am very fond of hotels with several floors; the more the merrier.

―――

It's time to reiterate what we've talked about. You've stumbled into the fifties while you weren't even looking, and you're in the second half of your life. The time to make change and prepare for the rest of your life is right now. Don't suffer the consequences of an unhealthy lifestyle later. There are enough uncontrollable possibilities which can happen to you, so don't add to life's unexpected problems by doing yourself in by eating junk and empty calories, being physically inactive, nonproductive, depressed and possibly lonely. Cut back or don't smoke, cut back or don't drink alcohol, don't consume large quantities of caffeine, switch to decaffeinated coffee if you crave your coffee, and don't live with long term stress.

Make a good night's sleep a habit, buy yourself a blood pressure machine, get your lipid profile checked, be productive. Exercise several times a week, warm up, cool down, and do some balancing tricks. If you need to lose a few pounds, DO IT. Hug loved ones and pet and walk your new dog. Prevent diabetes! You are or will be retired and you need to embrace your new found freedom by enjoying and exploring the outdoors, breathing fresh air, and geting some appropriate sun exposure.

Remember all the changes your aging body is going through in the transitional decade. Don't accelerate the aging process by doing the wrong things. All of us are not living in the future Star Trek generation where laboratory enhanced telomeres are going to come into play and somehow stop the time clock. After all, we are simply young people born earlier. Live correctly right now, and you will stay younger longer.

That's the *spirit*!

Appendix

Chapter 7 – Alcohol
***
AUDIT test
The AUDIT test is reprinted with permission from the World Health Organization.
AUDIT, Appendix B, page 31, Box 10
http://whqlibdoc.who.int/hq/2001WHO_MSD/MSB_01.6a.pdf
Notes: A Clinician's Guide for Helping Patients Who Drink Too Much
US Department of Health and Human Services

Chapter 9 – Dogs
A list of journals where you may find articles related to the health benefits from dogs:
Hypertension, Medical Journal of Australia, American Journal of Cardiology
American Journal of Transplantation, The Journal of Nervous and Mental Disease
American Journal of Occupation Therapy, Journal of Pediatric Nursing
People, Animals, Environment, Childhood Education
Journal of the Royal Society of Medicine, Memorial Sloan-Kettering Cancer Center,
Dept. of Social Work. Society for Research in Child Development
International Conference on Human-Animal Interactions, Journal of Social Psychology

Chapter 11 – Disorders

For more information about your heart, lipids and prevention of associated diseases, please refer to these credible sources:

American Heart Association – http://www.heart.org

Centers for Disease Control and Prevention – http://www.cdc.gov

Framingham Heart Study/Coronary Heart Disease Risk – http://www.framinghamheartstudy.org/risk/coronary.html

National Heart, Lung, and Blood Institute – http://www.nhlbi.nih.gov

About the Author

Barbara Ebel is a physician and writer. She attended University of Louisville medical school, University of Louisville residency program, and practiced in Louisville and Florida as a board-certified anesthesiologist. She doesn't presently practice anesthesia, but has used her primary care skills as a clinic volunteer physician and on a medical mission. She is a medical guest lecturer on topics ranging from physician suicide to Malignant Hyperthermia.

Doctor Barbara sprinkles credible medicine into the background of her novels and her operating room scenes shine, but her characters and plots take center stage. She has also written and illustrated a children's book series called *Chester the Chesapeake* about her therapy dog.

As an author, she is situated in the right spot for writing, nestled into a wildlife corridor in middle Tennessee with her husband and pets. She has lived up and down the East Coast and always enjoys being close to the Atlantic, the Gulf of Mexico, or lakes and rivers.

The following books are also written by Barbara Ebel and are available as paperbacks and eBooks:

Operation Neurosurgeon: *You never know… who's in the OR* (the first book in the Dr. Danny Tilson Novels, an excerpt is below)

Silent Fear: a Medical Mystery (the second book in the Dr. Danny Tilson Novels)

Collateral Circulation: a Medical Mystery (the third book in the Dr. Danny Tilson Novels)

Outcome, A Novel: *There's more than a hurricane coming...*

You may visit the author at her website: http://barbaraebel.weebly.com

Also written and illustrated by Barbara Ebel:

A children's book series about her loveable therapy dog:
Chester the Chesapeake Book One
Chester the Chesapeake Book Two: Summertime
Chester the Chesapeake Book Three: Wintertime
Chester the Chesapeake Book Four: My Brother Buck
Chester the Chesapeake Book Five: The Three Dogs of Christmas
The Chester the Chesapeake Trilogy (The Chester the Chesapeake Series) – eBook only
Visit Chester the Chesapeake and his books at:
http://dogbooksforchildren.weebly.com

Operation Neurosurgeon:

You never know ... who's in the OR

By Barbara Ebel, M.D.

A Dr. Danny Tilson Novel.

Chapter 1

- 2009 -

Through the desolate winter woods, she could see a run-down single story house. She firmly pressed the accelerator to climb the hilly, rutted road as pebbles kicked up from the gravel, pinging underneath her sedan. All around her, tall spindly trees stood without a quiver, the area still, quiet and remote. On this damp, cold February afternoon, she had come to conclude a deal with a man named Ray.

The road narrowed past the house, fading over the hill, but she veered slowly to the left, a barren area in front of the peeling house, where a dusty red pickup truck stood idle and a black plumaged vulture busily scavenged. Deliberately she left her belongings, clicked the lock on her car and walked to the front door. She threw the long end of her rust scarf behind her shoulder. The raptor grunted through his hooked beak as he flew off to the backwoods. The door opened before she knocked.

"Nobody visits a feller like me," the man said, smiling at her while adjusting his baseball cap, "unless we're buying and selling. You must be the lady with the book."

The tidily shaven man wore a salt and pepper colored beard and mustache and an open plaid cotton shirt with a tee shirt underneath. The boots peeking out from under his blue jeans had seen muddy days.

The woman smiled pleasantly at him and went in the front door empty handed. If the man had any furniture, she wasn't aware of it. Car parts lay strewn everywhere, which made her wonder if he slept in a bed.

Ray followed her glance. "You nearly can't find one of them no mores," he said, pointing to a charcoal-colored, elongated piece of vinyl plastic on the floor. She looked quizzically at him and shoved the woolen hat she'd been wearing into her pocket.

"It's an original 1984 Mercedes dashboard. See, the holes are for vents and the radio. Got a bite on that one from a teenager restoring his first car." She didn't seem interested though. She eyed the dust, in some spots thick as bread.

"Are you sure you have twelve-thousand dollars to pay for this?" she asked, unbuttoning her jacket.

"You come out thirty miles from Knoxville? That baby in your belly may need something," he said, pointing to her pregnancy. "You want a soda or something?"

"No, thank you," she said, grimacing at him.

"Oh, yeah. I got the money," he said. "All I got now to my name is seventy-five thousand dollars. I got ruint in Memphis. Was a part owner in a used car dealership. Went away for a little while and the other guy cleaned me out. Can't afford nothing like a lawyer to chase 'im down."

She tapped her foot.

"Anyhow, I won't bother yer with all that. I got a thing going good on eBay. I got a reputation, it ain't soiled. You can trust me, I give people what I tell them, whether I'm buying or selling."

A beagle-looking mutt crawled out from behind a car door. "Molly, your milk containers are dragging on the floor. Better get out to your pups," the man said, prodding her out the partially-closed door.

"You like dogs?" he asked.

"I suppose so."

"I got no use for people who don't care for dogs. Something not right about people like that."

The woman turned and followed the clumsy dog outside, grabbed a bag from the front seat, and came back in. She took out a book, opened the back cover, and handed him a folded piece of paper. *Certificate of Authenticity*, the man read, from a company in New Orleans, verifying the signature on the front page to be Albert Einstein's. He inverted his hand and wiggled his fingers, gesturing to her if he could hold the aged book.

"Where'd you say you got it?" He observed her carefully.

"It's been in the family for years. I took my precious belongings with me when I left New Orleans because of Hurricane Katrina. Since I lost my house there, I decided to stay in Tennessee. Now I'm selling my expensive things. I have to make ends meet, especially with a baby coming."

"Good thing you got this certificate with it then. Twelve-thousand dollars, we've got a deal."

He walked away to the back of the house while she held on to the physicist's 1920 publication. He came through the doorway with a stack of money and a brown paper bag. She nodded once when she finished counting the bills, so he handed her the empty bag.

"I still got your email address and phone number," he said. "I keep track of what goes and comes."

"You won't need them," she said and left abruptly.

He watched her back out and stood there until the car disappeared out of sight down the gray road.